GLOBAL
SERVICE-LEARNING
IN NURSING

Tamara H. McKinnon, MSN, RN
Joyce Fitzpatrick, PhD, MBA, RN, FAAN, FNAP
Editors

National League
for **Nursing**

National League for Nursing
61 Broadway
New York, NY 10006
212-363-5555 or 800-669-1656
www.nln.org

ISBN 978-1-934758-14-4

Cover Design by Brian Vigorita
Art Director, Laerdal Medical Corporation

Printed in the United States of America

Global Service-Learning in Nursing

Dedication

This book is dedicated to all partners in global service-learning who strive to make the world a more healthful and peaceful place.

List of Tables

List of Figures

Before it gained increasing notice in the nursing community, global service-learning (GSL) was a consuming passion of Tamara H. McKinnon. During our very first conversation, Tamara demonstrated a great deal of enthusiasm about her completed modules regarding developing and sustaining global service-learning programs. Over a 15-year period, Tamara researched questions about participants in these initiatives, reasons for their involvement, host sites, and outcomes of the experiences. For ease of evaluation and reduced frustration, she concluded that nursing education leaders could benefit from a standardized method to develop global service-learning programs. Therefore, this toolkit was written for nurse leaders thinking about developing a global service-learning experience or sustaining and strengthening current initiatives.

There are some who would argue that standardization means homogeneity. I respectfully disagree. Just as nursing education programs meet national accreditation criteria but retain the uniqueness of their own institutional culture, so it is with standards for global service-learning. To ensure a broad perspective, Tamara invited a number of authors – diverse in race, ethnicity, and thought – to contribute to this book.

Chapter 1 discusses seven basic best practice principles imperative for all GSL programs: compassion, curiosity, courage, collaboration, creativity, capacity building, and competence. The case study in this chapter clarifies these principles while highlighting ethical considerations relevant to global service-learning. It is around these principles that global service-learning programs can be standardized.

Chapter 2 offers a start toward a systematic theoretical approach to developing GSL partnerships, with an emphasis on systems theory and appreciative inquiry. Systems theory offers a means by which to capture the complexity of health and health care in a host community and build a framework for interventions. Appreciative inquiry emphasizes the strengths of communities in an effort to co-create sustainable interventions. Together, systems theory and appreciative inquiry can serve as the foundation for a new conceptualization of GSL that will help ensure consistency in planning and evaluation of programs, and meaningful goal setting.

Chapter 3 outlines four steps that can aid in developing and sustaining an effective global service-learning program in nursing education: planning, method, building relationships, and evaluation. Extensive and thorough planning leads to positive and effective implementation. Reasons for being involved in a host community are clarified, and capacity building is emphasized. Building relationships is highlighted as a key to success.

Perspectives from partners are reviewed in Chapters 4 through 8, where different individuals share insights and stories reflecting the point of view of different stakeholders in a GSL program. The topics covered include a comprehensive step-by-step guide to setting up a GSL program by the home institution (Chapter 4); the complementary roles of home institution faculty and administration (Chapter 5); the challenges faced by a host institution receiving international students (Chapter 6); the necessity of building a partnership between home and host (Chapter 7); and the role of student participants as program partners (Chapter 8). These chapters offer a wealth of useful information and observations, both small and large. Here readers will learn that planning for unplanned time is a key strategy helpful for networking, dealing with jetlag, and a host of other concerns. Here they will find a well-laid-out, clear delineation of faculty and administration responsibilities and guidance for how the two can work together to create a smooth-running program. Here, too, readers will discover how to provide appropriate resources for foreign students, and how to involve their own students in planning an international program.

Chapter 9 presents four exemplars, representing different experiences. One author teaches at an institution that has been running global service-learning programs for 35 years; she offers the benefit of her school's long and extensive experience. Another author helped develop a new global service-learning course. A third describes her experience as a nursing student who shadowed a registered nurse in Ireland; she was enlightened by the cultural immersion and began to appreciate the strengths of others. Finally, the fourth author describes how her passion for developing students as global citizens was not enough to get a GSL program running, despite her best efforts. As she found out, sometimes timing is everything – timing and support.

Chapter 10 is the outgrowth of Tamara's realization that despite a growing body of research on GSL, little is known about the extent or types of international service or study programs available in U.S. schools of nursing. To help fill this gap, Tamara developed a survey, with support from the National League for Nursing (NLN), to elicit baseline data on global service-learning experiences in nursing education programs. The results of the survey have been shared with the International Nursing Education Services and Accreditation (INESA), a joint task force of the National League for Nursing and the NLN Accrediting Commission. This chapter provides a brief overview of the survey's methods and analysis of its results, which will be published in fuller form elsewhere. And last but not least, Chapter 11 provides a list of global resources available to nurse educators and schools of nursing interested in strengthening or establishing a global service-learning program.

In Tamara's words, "This could be an exciting and important collaboration which will provide direction for current and future nurse leaders in global service learning." I agree with her without reserve.

Virginia W. Adams
Consultant, National League for Nursing
Inaugural Chair, International Council of Nurses Education Network

Global service-learning is a state of mind, a willingness to learn from others and to serve others no matter where they live. Global service-learning for nursing education requires a reframing of our understandings of "here" and "elsewhere." We are all part of the same universe of nurses, serving individuals, families, and communities in our hometowns and across the world. More importantly, global service-learning requires a commitment to learn from each other in the process of teaching others about our own beliefs, values, and understandings.

This book represents an assessment of where we are as nurse educators in developing programs of global service-learning. Nurse educators from a wide range of institutions share their insights about the successes and challenges of program development, implementation, and evaluation. There are undoubtedly a myriad of stories behind each partnership and project, for each time we develop a new global connection we learn so much about our partners and their culture. We create memories of others, of their strengths and limitations, of their struggles for health and wellness, and we conclude that we are more alike than different. And importantly, we learn about ourselves.

Each of our cultures strives for the best for its citizens. I remember fondly the nurses I have worked with in many countries. The nurses in Uganda were steadfast in their positive attitudes toward HIV care delivery, and committed to the values of social justice for those affected by the HIV pandemic. The nurses in Middle Eastern countries, who at the time I met them had only recently received access to ideas from the West, were most eager to share their perspectives on life and health in their societies. The nurses in South Korea, Taiwan, and Thailand, who had access to education at the graduate level, were developing their own skills to better the lives of others. I remember their faces and their names, but mostly I remember their stories, their dedication to improving the health of others they served.

While our models of health care delivery may be different, as nurses we are all oriented to providing the best possible care with the resources available – and we are fortunate to have the knowledge and skills to serve, and to transcend cultures and countries to serve others. The language "I am a nurse" speaks volumes to other nurses, and importantly, to individuals everywhere. The nursing bond is strong and powerful, and serves as the foundation for global service-learning programs such as those described in this book – a testimony to the worldwide service of nurses.

While many individuals contributed their work and their thoughts to the design, implementation, and production of this book, it is important to acknowledge the book's genesis. The idea was born of the passion and dedicated work of my co-editor, Tamara McKinnon, who had been envisioning such an undertaking for years. Tamara lives the spirit of global service-learning, taking every opportunity to expand her environment, to reach out to others who might share a perspective that would enlighten her own understandings. She is a constant student, learning from others formally and informally, to provide the greatest good for the students she teaches and ultimately for the individuals she serves. While this book is a product of her doctoral studies at Case Western Reserve University and a partnership developed with the National League for Nursing, it is more than that for Tamara, and hopefully for our readers.

The global service-learning model offers an excellent structure within which to enhance our participation in the global health care community. This book charts the course of our accomplishments thus far, and challenges us to stretch even more.

Joyce J. Fitzpatrick, Co-editor

Every author involved in this work demonstrates a passion for global service-learning. Each individual and team contributed selflessly to the collaborative effort, sharing generously their expertise and experiences. Their enthusiasm, commitment, and professionalism are making a difference in global health.

The National League for Nursing has provided every conceivable means of support to facilitate the development of this book. M. Elaine Tagliareni, Virginia W. Adams, Janice Brewington, Justine Fitzgerald, and Meira Ben-Gad have been particularly helpful in developing the text. Joyce J. Fitzpatrick's unwavering confidence that people can accomplish absolutely anything they set their mind to is remarkable. This book was made possible by Joyce's amazing ability to establish connections between individuals whose combined efforts can move mountains.

I owe a debt of gratitude to Joyce and others who have supported and mentored me in my career, particularly Carol Huston, Jayne Cohen, Anne Farrier, and Marianne Hultgren. Gerard M. Fealy and Angela M. McNelis are the most gracious writing partners one could hope for.

I would like to thank my students for reminding me what an honor it is to be a nurse, and my 'Amigas' for sharing insights and waves. Most importantly, I would like to acknowledge my husband Dave and our sons Aaron and Lucas, who are a constant source of love and support.

Tamara H. McKinnon

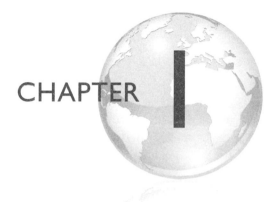

CHAPTER 1

Core Principles for Developing Global Service-Learning Programs in Nursing*

Tamara H. McKinnon
Gerard M. Fealy

*Reprinted with permission from the National League for Nursing

McKinnon, T. H. and Fealy, G. (2011). Core concepts for developing global service-learning programs in nursing. *Nursing Education Perspectives, 32*(2), 95-101.

Service-learning gives nursing students and practicing nurses opportunities to learn and grow as nurses while serving communities and populations in deliberate and tangible ways. In its many forms, service-learning offers a range of experiences and opportunities that can help students develop a repertoire of skills for delivering effective health care, while building cultural competence and fostering a sense of civic responsibility. Global service-learning (GSL) can involve international campus-community partnerships and initiatives in diverse communities closer to home. Through global service-learning, nursing can strengthen its role in promoting global health by helping vulnerable and marginalized communities both at home and around the world further their own capacity for growth and development.

Ultimately, the success of GSL depends on good planning based on sound, best-practice principles. The principles discussed in this article are distilled from an extensive body of literature and are based on the Seven Cs of Best Practice: Compassion, Curiosity, Courage, Collaboration, Creativity, Capacity Building, and Competence (see Figure 1-1). The Seven Cs have been shown to foster ethical and compassionate learning experiences, local or global, and are key to the successful development of effective and sustainable service-learning programs.

Figure 1.1
Seven Cs of Global Service-Learning

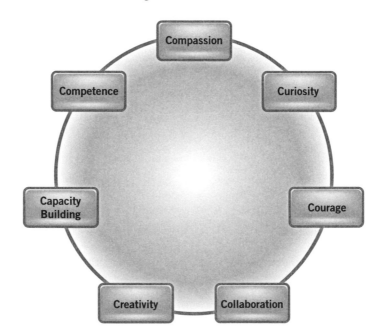

The Goals and Conceptual Basis of Service-Learning

As an action-oriented pedagogical approach, service-learning enables students to engage in real-world, community-focused activities that contribute in meaningful ways to their learning (Seifer, 1998) and their academic and social development (Simpson, 1998). Service-learning is predicated on the view that classroom learning alone cannot provide students with the sorts of experiences that enable them to develop citizenship and civic responsibility. For nursing students at the undergraduate and graduate levels, service-learning contributes to their preparation for the roles of nurse and citizen (Nokes, Nickitas, Keida, & Neville, 2005) and helps them develop an understanding of the cultural and health care contexts in which their nursing skills may be deployed (Eyler, 2002).

The concept of service-learning developed from broad ideas about the role and social relevance of the university, including the idea that the university is responsible for inculcating in students a sense of civic responsibility, not just knowledge and skills. Service-learning also emerged from ideas about pedagogy, including Dewey's belief that learning directed toward the welfare of others can promote both academic and social development (Simpson, 1998) and is more meaningful if it takes place in real-world settings (Seifer, 1998).

Bringle and Hatcher (1996) proposed that service-learning falls on a continuum between charitable community service and experiential learning in professional training. The term is not synonymous with charity or volunteerism, and equally not with field studies or mandatory placements in a practicum (McKinnon et al., 2009). By offering their knowledge, skills, and time, students serve a community through service actions, and, in turn, learn new context-relevant knowledge and skills (Sinclair & Zinger, 2008). Specific academic goals and objectives of service activities are linked in a deliberate way to the service experience (Farley, 2003).

In 2007, the nursing honor society Sigma Theta Tau International (STTI) established an International Service-Learning Task Force (ISLTF), with members from across the globe. The ISLTF examined international service-learning programs and identified strategies that STTI could use to create its own meaningful international service-learning program. The group adopted a definition of service-learning as a process that "integrates community service with academic study to meet a community need and enrich student learning by providing planned community-based activities that provide students with meaningful and explicit learning" (McKinnon et al., 2009). This definition, representing the consensus position of ISLTF members, accounts for variations in understandings of service-learning across countries and cultures.

While incorporating elements of experiential learning, service-learning can encompass a range of activities and outcomes, including community service, civic engagement, citizenship, social responsibility, and cultural competence. The latter is the concept that is most frequently cited as a desirable outcome of global service-learning. Cultural competence is defined by Campinah-Bacote (2002) as "the integration of cultural awareness, cultural knowledge, cultural skill, cultural encounters, and cultural desire" (p. 181). Campinah-Bacote contends that these various constructs are interdependent and must be experienced or expressed in the encounter between the health care provider and the client or community. There is a direct relationship between the level of competence of health care providers and their ability to provide culturally responsive health care services. Building on Campinah-Bacote's definition, cultural competence in nursing consists of knowing oneself first and then being interested in, becoming knowledgeable about, and developing the skills needed to provide relevant and meaningful nursing care to members of various cultural groups. Service-learning programs offer students opportunities to become immersed in another culture and develop the skills necessary to provide culturally competent care (Amerson, 2010).

Why Core Principles Are Needed

Cultural competence is achieved at a number of levels: the individual, community, organization, and society (Calvillo et al., 2009). For the community, benefits derive from meeting particular needs for health care and community development and the promotion of social justice. Learner and community outcomes will only be achieved if the process of delivering a service is built on sound principles that include mutuality, reciprocity, and respect. Partnership is a core value of service-learning. Through partnership, educational institutions and communities can work together to overcome complex community and social problems.

With the world growing increasingly smaller, having a corps of nurses who are committed to providing relevant and appropriate patient care to diverse communities is a social and moral imperative. Indeed, nursing has a remarkable history of developing GSL programs (Riner & Becklenberg, 2001) that involve cross-cultural and international immersion experiences and health care delivery, mainly in developing countries. Examples include health clinics run by U.S. nurses and doctors in a poor community in Kingston, Jamaica (Walsh, 2004), and immersion placements in developing countries such as Ecuador (Bentley & Ellison, 2007) and Nicaragua (Kollar & Ailinger, 2002; Riner & Becklenberg, 2001). But the GSL imperative has also produced programs run by and for nurses locally. In the United States, there are a myriad of programs in which nurses work to advance global health with diverse populations in both rural and urban settings. Examples of such initiatives include health care programs among low-income families (Hamner, Wilder, & Byrd, 2007) and community-dwelling seniors (Lutz, Herrick, & Lehman, 2001), developmental screening services for at-risk youth (Kushto-Rees,

Maguire, Silbert-Flagg, Immelt, & Shaefer, 2007), a health needs assessment service in a homeless family shelter (Hunt & Swiggum, 2007), a school health service for low-income neighborhood grade school children (Lough, 1999), and a schools-based adolescent health promotion program for economically disadvantaged black and Hispanic communities (Juhn et al., 1998).

Irrespective of the type of service activity, all programs should share a set of unifying principles that offer a means of standardizing program development at the macro level. It is critical that nursing articulate its unique contribution to global health and community development and its place in the field of global health through global service-learning. It is also important to note that while global service-learning opportunities are available to practicing nurses as well as students, all participants in GSL programs are, in actuality, students.

The Seven Cs of Program Development

The core principles for global service-learning in nursing are offered here to provide nurse faculty and program planners with a basis for best practice in program development. The articulation of core principles for GSL provides for consistency across programs while allowing individual programs to maintain their uniqueness at the level of program content and focus. Incorporating these principles provides for enhanced communication among programs, greater opportunity for collaborative research, and consistency of evaluation criteria. It also allows nursing to articulate its distinct role in global health.

In what follows we offer a brief overview of each of the seven principles, along with a case study exemplar that unfolds as each principle is discussed.

Compassion. Compassion provides the impetus for change and is a key motivator for establishing a GSL program. The journey begins with empathy, friendship, and caring for the clients and communities who will benefit when nurses are impelled by a dedication to justice in health care provision. The result is dedication to creating a generation of nurses who possess a global perspective on health care.

Many nurses are motivated by the desire to gain a global understanding of health care in their work, as well as to develop new skills and capabilities through community service. Kelley, Connor, Kun, and Salmon (2008) point out that social responsibility is strongly linked to the values held by the health professions in general and by the nursing profession in particular. As they put it "the underlying constructs of social responsibility are woven into the fabric of nursing's history and its codes of ethics and practice" (p. 4). The principle of social responsibility is closely linked with service-learning, and service-learning has been demonstrated to enhance civic responsibility (Reising et al., 2008).

Gloria is a clinical instructor of public health in a school of nursing in Colorado. Several years ago, she attended a seminar hosted by her institution on the topic of international nonprofit organizations. The guest speaker, Michael, represented a nongovernmental organization (NGO) working in a host community in a developing country. The NGO's mission is to provide microloans to individuals with the goal of economic development. Michael spoke eloquently about the challenges and rewards of working with community members. He shared stories of how the work of his organization had transformed individuals, families, and communities. He also recounted heartbreaking stories of unmet needs, including health care needs, experienced by the host community.

Months later, Gloria continued to find herself thinking of those who had been helped by the NGO, as well as the health issues faced by the host community. Building on her lifelong passion for providing her students with meaningful and challenging clinical experiences, her compassion led her to make a commitment to finding a way to help by developing a global service-learning program at her school.

Curiosity. Although difficult to define and measure, curiosity is critical to the development of a GSL program. The process of exploring ways to create opportunities for students can lead to innovative approaches to program development. Curiosity about other cultures and issues in global health, as well as a keen interest in the learning needs of program participants, are both critical. Identification of areas that are interesting and exciting to the program leader is essential to engendering the energy and enthusiasm needed to sustain a program.

Wehling (2008) writes that "by venturing into the community, students see beyond the cultural walls that often divide neighborhoods, and they also make connections between economics, anthropology, history, political science, and other disciplines" (p. 294). The process can satisfy students' quest for new knowledge and understandings of global health and is itself grounded in curiosity.

Gloria became curious about how she might go about working with her students to provide services to the community. She was also interested in learning more about the host community, specifically their health needs and resources. Motivated by questions such as "What could I possibly do?" and "What would my role be?" she began researching the concept of GSL. She also inquired about her school's relationship with Michael's organization and initiated discussions with her students about their interest in GSL and serving a disadvantaged community. The more Gloria researched the matter, the stronger grew her desire to identify a means of addressing the health care needs of the community through GSL.

Courage. There is no template for GSL program development. Program leaders, partners, and participants must possess the courage to embark on a long and often challenging journey. Being a strong and effective program leader requires willingness and an ability to lead by example. The courageous leader is one who is completely committed to the process and willing to trust his or her instincts in taking the initial requisite steps in program development.

Participants must also exhibit courage, since they are embarking on a journey into unfamiliar territory. Recognizing that there will likely be challenges ahead, they can take the risk of participating in a program with the confidence that it will bring them personal and professional rewards.

In making a long-term commitment to service-learning, institutions also require courage. GSL programs challenge institutions to support the application of knowledge in real-world settings and to promote civic and social responsibility among students (McKinnon et al., 2009). In this, service-learning represents the "teaching dimension of the scholarship of engagement" (Zlotkowski, 2007). Yet embarking on this path can be threatening to institutions. Cohen and Milone-Nuzzo (2001) write that service-learning can give rise to institutional change in that it leads to questioning about common practices of both the service agency and the educational institution.

Gloria never thought this would be a simple undertaking, but she was astonished to realize the complexity of the task ahead. Since there was no precedent for a GSL program at her school of nursing, her initial inquiries about program development were met with resistance by her colleagues and her dean. The concept of GSL was foreign to them, they felt that too little was known about the subject, and they encouraged Gloria to stick with the status quo.

Nevertheless, Gloria was not dissuaded. Her passion for developing a GSL program was rooted in compassion for a community in need, along with her newly acquired knowledge regarding the positive outcomes of such programs for students. She presented her case eloquently and convincingly to the dean and was granted approval to develop a program offering GSL to a small group of students. Gloria then contacted Michael, who was thrilled at the prospect of developing a relationship with the school of nursing. Convinced that maintaining the status quo was simply not an ethical course of action, Gloria had taken the first concrete steps toward developing a GSL program.

Collaboration. The goal of service-learning is the creation of dynamic partnerships between educational institutions and communities, in which the needs of program participants and the communities that they serve are of equal importance (Peterson & Schaffer, 1999). Indeed, it might be said that the partners in a GSL program are the host community, the home institution, and the program participants. The partnership must be established on the basis of negotiations between the host community and home institution regarding key program structures and processes, such as who controls access to resources, the relative contributions of staff, and the pattern and flow of relationships (Foss, Bonaiuto, Johnson, & Moreland, 2003). Community-Campus Partnerships for Health (CCPH), a nonprofit organization based at the University of Washington, outlines 10 principles of good community-campus partnerships (CCPH, 2011). For example: a) The relationship between partners is characterized by mutual trust, respect, genuineness, and commitment. b) The partnership balances power among partners and enables resources to be shared. c) Principles and processes for the partnership are established with the input and agreement of all partners.

Just as community engagement is a core academic and scholarly activity (Holland, Gelmon, & Gelmon, 1998), academic-civic partnerships represent a core educational value (Zlotkowski, 2007). Partnership is the ethical and professional responsibility of all GSL programs, and collaboration is the practical expression of commitment to the partnership.

Some programs insinuate themselves into a community, provide a service, and then leave that community. This approach to international work is unethical and often leaves the community reluctant to pursue future global partnerships, particularly when vulnerable communities are involved. Community engagement needs faculty leaders and mentors who will sustain academic-community partnership activities over time and who will integrate engagement into their overall scholarly agenda (Holland et al., 1998). In addition, reciprocal exchanges reflect a high level of collaboration and are becoming increasingly popular.

Examples of collaborative endeavors include engaging in joint research and publications, and sharing resources efficiently and wisely across programs. Indeed, efficient sharing of resources is a hallmark of an ethical GSL program, and enables both academic institutions and community agencies to maximize limited resources (Foss et al., 2003).

Collaboration requires hard work and coalition building. It can be considered in terms of a number of steps: a) identifying community leaders and a primary liaison person; b) exploring community priorities; c) identifying community resources and competencies; d) mutual goal setting; e) establishing and maintaining open, ongoing communication; and (f) where relevant, producing joint research and publications.

Once the decision had been made to move forward, Gloria realized that she needed to clarify the role and relationship of each partner in the GSL program: her institution and herself as its representative; the host community; and the student participants. Her role and that of her institution were clear. She would be the program leader for a project offering GSL for school of nursing credit for a small group of senior-level students over the summer term.

Gloria researched the role of students in GSL programs in nursing and other disciples and developed a curriculum that included pre- and post-immersion training for students. She found that the greatest challenge was establishing a collaborative relationship with the host community. Michael was instrumental in connecting Gloria with leaders in the community, particularly those involved in the provision of health care. She began communicating directly with these key individuals and presented the possibility of establishing a GSL initiative. Her communication focused on establishing a clear sense of the community's goals and needs around health and the resources in place to initiate and sustain change.

Gloria had read accounts of "parachute" programs, which were developed with good intentions but whose results were disastrous. Determined to avoid such missteps, Gloria established and maintained active, open communication with community leaders. Her assessment was conducted through these individuals as well as through research on the host community's culture, beliefs, and health practices. Local health care organizations provided her with valuable information. In addition, to ensure that planned program interventions were realistic, she paid particular attention to the community's resources and infrastructure.

Gloria's efforts paid off. She was invited by the director of a small clinic to bring a group of students the following year. Over the course of the year, Gloria worked with the clinic director to identify mutually agreed upon realistic and sustainable goals for the program.

Creativity. Like curiosity, creativity is difficult to define and difficult to measure. Yet creativity fuels effective program development and is an important principle for program planners, both at the macro level, when partnerships are sought and formed, and at the micro level of service provision and in the conduct of pedagogical activities associated with the service. GSL programs provide many opportunities for innovation and are especially appropriate for original ideas that link education and a commitment to community service, either locally or globally. Such programs can be fertile ground for the testing of new and innovative approaches to preparatory and continuing education for nurses.

The innovative use of technology is one way program developers can apply creative thinking to suggest new approaches to old problems in curriculum design and instruction. Sigma Theta Tau's *Vision 2020* encourages program developers to design methods that foster global community building through education, communication and technology innovations, such as creating an open electronic knowledge repository (STTI, 2007). The result will be vibrant and meaningful GSL programs that are attuned to innovations and ideas from other programs around the world while remaining responsive to the culture and unique characteristics of the host community. Creativity in program development can help build novel learning experiences for GLS program participants and is a feature of the development of what Newman (2008) refers to as *participatory knowledge.*

Without a template for program development, Gloria identified constraints and requirements of the program and then allowed her creativity to take over. In many ways this was liberating for her. She was able to imagine the vibrant and meaningful program that she knew each partner was searching for. In the process of researching a plan for GSL development, Gloria realized that she was practicing innovative teaching principles. Reading Benner's recent work (Benner, Sutphen, Leonard, & Day, 2010) and thinking about theories such as Appreciative Inquiry were particularly instructional during this phase of program development.

One novel approach Gloria decided upon involved the use of technology. She partnered with a fellow faculty member who would be teaching a lecture course over the summer and developed a plan to have students in the GSL program interact online with students working in the classroom. The GSL students would craft questions for those at the home institution, and the groups would then work together to develop an appropriate plan of action. Other methods of innovative teaching involved the use of social networking and blogging prior to the program and continuing into orientation for future participants. Social media etiquette was included in the orientation for students.

Gloria worked with her primary liaison in the host community to plan a day of orientation for the students upon their arrival. Local experts on topics such as the area's culture, music, and food would teach classes.

Realizing that the cost of the program was financially burdensome for many students, Gloria led the group in a series of fundraising activities. These were productive, both in terms of raising funds and in developing a sense of fellowship among participants. The fundraising events provided a public relations opportunity for the GSL program, and the school of nursing received positive feedback from university leaders.

Capacity Building. In developing humanitarian health projects, health care workers need to avoid interventions that cultivate a dependent relationship (Walsh, 2004). The focus should be on helping the host community build the necessary capacity to establish its own resources for health care and community development, thereby empowering the community and increasing its capacity for growth (Kidder, 2004). To accomplish this, the institutional-community partnership should be based not only on the host community's needs for health improvement, but on its identified strengths and assets (CCPH, 2011).

Capacity building is therefore part of ethical program development. Effective GSL programs lead to active, synergistic, and sustainable relationships between program participants and communities. The goal of capacity building is to continuously improve the partnership and its outcomes, to the point where the home and host communities mutually benefit without either relying on the other (CCPH, 2011).

After a year of planning, Gloria and her group of students were on the airplane, ready to embark. She was feeling excited and a bit anxious but was confident that the preparation she had done would lead to the desired outcomes. The emphasis on building capacity of all partners was at the forefront of each step of the planning process. Her research on the resources and capacities of the host community, along with the goal setting and planning she had done in communication with community leaders, increased her confidence. It was interesting to Gloria that as the plane waited to take off, her thoughts were on another journey in the future, when the community's capacity would be such that she would be leading students on another program somewhere else.

Competence: *Core Principles as Building Blocks to Research.* As our case study illustrates, the application of the seven core principles is a sequential process; each step leads naturally to the next. While substantiation from the literature is offered in support of each individual step, evidenced-based research is needed to determine if the overall effects of implementing these steps leads to meaningful GSL programs. At the time of writing, the National League for Nursing was conducting research on the extent to which schools of nursing are involved in GSL. The results of this research should provide nursing with baseline information with which to develop further studies on the development and effectiveness of GSL programs.

According to Barrett and Fry (2008), inquiry is intervention. By asking what approaches should be taken to standardize GSL programs in nursing, we are moving forward on a path toward creative and meaningful solutions to this question.

In order to add to the body of evidence-based research on the topic of GSL, it is important to identify means of measuring the competencies of all three partners. This process should involve longitudinal measurement of the cultural competence, civic engagement, and leadership skills of participants.

Taking a deep breath, Gloria watched as her students were picked up from the airport upon their return from the first GSL program. Gloria reflected on the commitment she had made a year before to explore and measure ways in which the GSL program could lead to increased competence on the part of all participants. Based on her exit interview with liaisons from the host community, it was evident that they were on target with previously established steps toward achieving self-articulated long-range goals. Student competence would be measured following the immersion, using standardized tools that had also been used during the preprogram orientation. These results would guide Gloria's future and would also contribute to the growing body of knowledge on outcomes of GSL for participants.

Gloria considered the path her life had taken over the previous year. Her confidence was high and she knew that she had developed valuable skills in the area of GSL program development. She thought about how far she had come, and how far she had yet to go. Gloria smiled, knowing that she was up for the challenge.

Conclusion

Global service-learning offers nursing an opportunity to develop its role in promoting global health and enabling global communities, especially vulnerable and marginalized communities, to develop their own capacity for growth and development. However, GSL requires proper planning, based on sound best-practice principles. The seven key principles that we have outlined here – compassion, curiosity, courage, collaboration, creativity, capacity building, and competence – form the basis for ethically sound program development, offer a means of standardizing program development, and can serve as a foundation for developing criteria by which to evaluate a program's success.

References

Amerson, R. (2010). The impact of service-learning on cultural competence. *Nursing Education Perspectives, 31*(1), 18–22.

Barrett, F., & Fry, R. (2008). *Appreciative inquiry: A positive approach to building cooperative capacity.* Chagrin Falls, OH: Taos Institute Publications.

Benner, P., Sutphen, M., Leonard, V., & Day, L. (2010). *Educating nurses: A call for radical transformation.* San Francisco, CA: Jossey-Bass.

Bentley, R., & Ellison, K. J. (2007) Increasing cultural competence in nursing through international service-learning experiences. *Nurse Educator, 32*(5), 207–211. doi:10.1097/01.NNE.0000289385.14007.b4

Bringle, R. G., & Hatcher J. A. (1996). Implementing service-learning in higher education *Journal of Higher Education, 67*(2), 221–239. doi:10.2307/2943981

Calvillo, E., Clark, L., Ballantyne, J. E., Pacquiao, D., Purnell. L. D., & Villarruel, A. M. (2009). Cultural competency in baccalaureate nursing education. *Journal of Transcultural Nursing, 20*(2), 137–145. doi:10.1177/1043659608330354

Campinah-Bacote, J. (2002). The process of cultural competence in the delivery of healthcare services: A model of care. *Journal of Transcultural Nursing, 13*(3), 181–184. doi:10.1177/10459602013003003

Cohen, S. S., & Milone-Nuzzo, P. (2001). Advancing health policy in nursing education through service-learning. *Advances in Nursing Science, 23*(3): 28–40. Retrieved from http://journals.lww.com/advancesinnursingscience/toc/2001/03000

Community-Campus Partnerships for Health (2010). *Principles of good community-campus partnerships.* Retrieved from www.ccph.info

Eyler, J. (2002) Reflecting on service: Helping nursing students get the most from service-learning. *Journal of Nursing Education, 4*, 453–456. doi:10.1111/1540-4560.00274

Farley, C. L. (2003). Service-learning: Applications in midwifery education. *Journal of Midwifery and Women's Health, 48*(6), 444–448. doi:10.1016/S1526-9523(03)00309-X

Foss, G. F., Bonaiuto, M. M., Johnson, S. Z., & Moreland D. M. (2003). Using Polvika's model to create a service-learning partnership. *Journal of School Health, 73*(8), 305–320. doi:10.1111/j.1746-1561.2003.tb06587.x

Hamner, J. B., Wilder, B., & Byrd, L. (2007) Lessons learned. Integrating a service learning community-based partnership into the curriculum. *Nursing Outlook 55*(2), 106–110. doi:10.1016/j.outlook.2007.01.008

Holland, B., & Gelmon, S., & Gelmon, S. B. (1998). The state of the 'engaged campus': What we have learned about building and sustaining university-community partnerships. *American Association of Higher Education Bulletin, 51*(2), 3–6.

Hunt, R. J., & Swiggum, P. (2007). Being in another world: Transcultural student experiences using service learning with families who are homeless. *Journal of Iranscultural Nursing, 18*(2), 167–174. doi: 10.1177/1043659606298614

Juhn, G., Tang, J., Pressens, P., Grant, U., Johnson, N. & Murray, H. (1998). Community learning: The reach for health nursing program-middle collaboration. *Journal of Nursing Education, 38*(5), 215–221.

Kelley, M., Connor, A., Kun, K. E., &Salmon, M. E. (2008). Social responsibility: Conceptualization and embodiment in a school of nursing. *International Journal of Nursing Education Scholarship, 5*(1), 1–16. doi:10.2202/1548-923X.1607

Kidder, T. (2004). *Mountains beyond mountains: The quest of Dr. Paul Farmer, a man who would cure the world.* New York: Random House.

Kollar, S. J., & Ailinger, R. L. (2002). International clinical experiences: Long term impact on students, *Nurse Educator, 27*(1) 28–31. doi:10.1097/00006223-200201000-00016

Kushto-Reese, K. C., Maguire, M. C., Silbert-Flagg, J. A., Immelt, S., & Shaefer, S. J. M. (2007). Developing community partnerships in nursing education for children's health. *Nursing Outlook, 55*(2), 85–94. doi:10.1016/j.outlook.2006.12.004

Lough, M. A. (1999). An academic-community partnership: A model of service and education. *Journal of Community Health Nursing, 16*(3), 137–149. doi:10.1207/S15327655JCHN1603_1

Lutz, J., Herrick, C. A., & Lehman, B. B. (2001). Community partnership: A school of nursing creates nursing centers for older adults. *Nursing and Health Care Perspectives, 22*(1), 26–29.

McKinnon, T., Bourgeois, S., DeNatale, M. L., Fealy, G. M., Gardner, J., Nickitas, D.,... Solomon-Middleton, L. (2009). *Final report of the International Service-Learning Task Force.* Indianapolis, IN: Sigma Theta Tau International.

Newman, M. (2008). *Transforming presence: The difference that nursing makes.* Philadelphia: FA Davis Company.

Nokes, K., Nickitas, D., Keida, R., & Neville, S. (2005). Does service-learning increase cultural competency, critical thinking, and civic engagement? *Journal of Nursing Education, 44*(2), 65–70. Retrieved from http://www.journalofnursingeducation.com/showAbst.asp?thing=34959

Norbeck, J., Connolly, C., & Koerner, J. (Eds.). (1998). *Caring and community concepts and models for service-learning in nursing.* Washington, DC: American Association for Higher Education.

Peterson, S., & Schaffer, M. (1999). Service-learning: A strategy to develop group collaboration and research skills. *Journal of Nursing Education, 38*(5), 208–214.

Reising, D, L., Shea, R. A., Allen, P. N., Laux, M. M., Hansel, D., & Watts, P. A. (2008). Using service-learning to develop health promotion and research skills in nursing students. *International Journal of Nursing Education Scholarship, 5*(1)., Article 29. doi:10.2202/1548-923X.1590

Riner, M. E., & Becklenberg, A. (2001). Partnering with a sister city organization for an international service-learning experience. *Journal of Transcultural Nursing, 12*(3), 234–240. doi:10.1177/104365960101200308

Seifer, S. D. (1998). Service-learning: Community-campus partnerships for health professions education. *Academic Medicine, 73*(3), 273–277. doi:10.1097/00001888-199803000-00015

Sigma Theta Tau International. (2010). *Vision 2020.* Indianapolis IN: Author. Retrieved from www.nursingsociety.org/aboutus/CalltoAction/Documents/Vision2020ExecutiveSummary.pdf

Simpson, J. (1998) Extension is not just service, but service-learning is important to extension. *Journal of Extension, 36*(5). Retrieved from http://www.joe.org/joe/1998october/comm1.html

Sinclair, A., & Zinger, L. (2008). Service-learning in nutrition education. *Academic Exchange Quarterly, 12*(3), 4117–4118. doi:10.1016/j.jada.2008.06.170

Walsh, D. S. (2004). A framework for short-term humanitarian health care projects. *International Nursing Review, 51*(1), 23–26. doi:10.1111/j.1466-7657.2003.00203.x

Wehling, S. (2008). Cross-cultural competency through service-learning. *Journal of Community Practice, 16*(3), 293–315. doi:10.1080/10705420802255080

Zlotkowski, E. (2007). The case for service-learning. In L. McIlraith & I. MacLabhrainn (Eds.), *Higher education and civic engagement: International perspectives* (pp. 37–52). Burlington, VT: Ashgate.

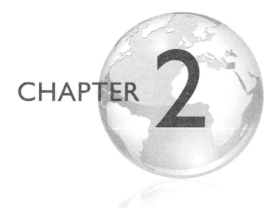

CHAPTER 2

A Theoretical Approach to Developing Global Service-Learning Partnerships

Virginia W. Adams

At this moment in time, nurses and nursing students around the world are participating in many scores of global service-learning initiatives aimed at advancing the health of developing populations. Partnerships and collaborations have been formed; institutes have been created; and students embark upon travel to far-flung places with the goal of helping improve the health of people in a host community. Often, before arrival, participants and program leaders have identified a problem in a host community that needs to be solved. Sometimes, they enter the international arena with the idea of presenting the best possible intervention to resolve problems, without an appreciation of the strengths that exist within the community or culture. In other words, they possess a notion of change and intervention based on their own interpretation of the needs of the host community. Such prescriptive approaches are often met with resistance.

A systematic theoretical approach will strengthen global service-learning experiences by reducing disparities in procedure and perspective among programs. Such an approach will make it more likely that nurse educators and learners will collect accurate data, analyze it in a meaningful way, and design programs of maximum benefit to the host community, educators, and learners. Moreover, host communities benefit from continuity in planning interventions. Without a theoretical framework, planning is inconsistent, evaluation is flawed, and goal setting becomes a moving target. Under such conditions, efforts made in advancing the health of the host population are less likely to be sustained.

This chapter considers general systems theory and the methodology of appreciative inquiry as frameworks for a systematic theoretical approach to global service-learning. General systems theory deals with the interactions and relationships among individuals in an organization, community, or other structured unit. Appreciative inquiry is an organizational development method that focuses on enlisting all parts of a system to identify strengths and build capacity within it. Together, systems theory and appreciative inquiry offer a model for a global service-learning approach that sees people both as whole and unique individuals, and within the context of the larger patterns of their lives. This model can serve as a foundation for designing global service-learning programs that will ensure long-term strength for global health systems.

Systems Theory

A systems theory approach entails understanding how the elements of a system influence one another to produce a whole that is greater than the sum of the parts. A system is a vast web of linkages and interactions, where the slightest intervention in one part affects those elements linked to it and, through them, the system as a whole. Systems thinking offers an approach to problem solving that views "problems" within the context of the larger system. In terms of health systems – which are complex on the local and national levels, let alone on the global front – systems theory can offer a methodical approach to unfolding complicated questions into more easily grasped smaller ones. As de Savigny and Adam (2009) put it, "systems thinking has huge and untapped potential, first in deciphering the complexity of an entire health system, and then in applying this understanding further to design and evaluate interventions that improve health and health equity" (p. 19).

A health system consists of all the interacting organizations, institutions, resources, and people whose primary purpose is to improve health. The World Health Organization has identified six subsystems, or building blocks, in health systems: service delivery, health workforce, health information, medical technologies, health financing, and leadership and governance (de Savigny & Adam, 2009). Each subsystem functions as a system on its own and as part of the larger health system. Designing an effective service-learning intervention requires understanding the relationships among these building blocks. Further, giving representatives from all the building blocks input into the design of an intervention can help ensure that the designers understand the intervention's likely impact on the entire system, and ensure support for the intervention from those who will be affected by it.

In this regard, when designing an intervention, assessing the openness of the system at issue is important. A system is viewed as open when inputs and outputs from both subsystems and supra-systems are free-flowing and pass through boundaries. In the context of systems theory, inputs are anything put into the system, and outputs are the information or outcome produced by the specific input. In the case of health care, inputs might be a new piece of diagnostic equipment or a process change, and the corresponding outputs would be the new diagnostic procedure or improvements in patient outcomes. When there is limited exchange of inputs and outputs, the system is viewed as closed. A closed system might be one in which, for example, the health providers in different communities do not share information on patients with infectious diseases, thus putting other communities and individuals at risk. A closed system may be inflexible, or may be set up to maintain boundaries or keep decision-making in a few hands. This is but one of the potential issues that can make it difficult to develop a sustainable intervention.

Designing a global service-learning program thus requires a close understanding of patterns among all the players, near and far, involved in health provision to a community. These patterns and relationships include those between subsystems or components belonging to varied disciplines, from medical technology down to communications and transportation. They also include relationships among individuals, within families, and between communities.

Among the many critical concepts relevant to service-learning – such as cultural proficiency, globalization, and partnership – the notion of partnership stands out.

Partnership implies that leaders and learners work together to achieve mutually agreed upon goals, through dialogue and open communication. The Center for the Advancement of Collaborative Strategies in Health, a research and resource center at the New York Academy of Medicine, expresses it this way: "In order to foster synergy, the leadership of a partnership needs to run a collaborative process that builds relationships and promotes meaningful discourse among different kinds of participants and helps partners create something new and valuable together" (Lasker & Weiss, 2002).

In short, the success of population-focused practice – i.e., health care aimed at improving the health of communities (Stanhope & Lancaster, 2010) – depends upon the strength of a collaborative effort involving many disciplines, the community, and the dynamic interactions between people and their environment, all intertwined and interdependent. For some people, this knowledge that any service-learning experience is but a small element in a larger system is liberating and a source of confidence. However, although a person's experience in one system is portable, the elements in the next system will operate differently.

Importantly, application of a systems theory approach does not mean that all questions will be answered, or – crucially – that there is one right answer to difficult questions. Sword, Reutter, Meagher-Stewart, and Rideout (2004) report on how Canadian baccalaureate students used service-learning experiences to understand poverty from the perspective of people living in those circumstances. For some of the students, the experience challenged their previous belief that poverty was an outcome of personal choices; they were influenced by their service-learning experience to focus more on system-wide, structural factors. Yet other students remained firm in the belief that people are responsible for the circumstances in which they live. Ultimately, the answer probably lies somewhere in between. Poverty is one part of a complex economic system that is linked to other large systems such as education and health. Systems theory offers a framework within which learners can examine those connections, clarifying the important questions if not necessarily providing answers.

Appreciative Inquiry

Appreciative inquiry (AI) is a philosophy that holds that it is possible to bring about change in large systems by capitalizing on the strengths of the system's components. Cooperrider and Srivastva (1987) are credited with coining the term appreciative inquiry and introducing it into the field of management. In Cooperrider's terms, AI is a theory of "non-deficit positive change" (Cooperrider & Sekerka, 2003), as contrasted with a problem solving or deficit-based philosophy. As Cooperrider (2010) put it, "What we appreciate (seeing value), appreciates (increases in value)." From a systems perspective, AI involves asking questions about what is right with the system rather than what is wrong, looking for the conditions under which people, organizations, and communities are most effective and most capable. Inherent in appreciative inquiry is a strategy of asking questions that evoke positive emotions. Evidence suggests that AI has been effective in a variety of settings. For instance, AI practitioners have brought together representatives from the world's chief religions in dialogue and mutual collaboration, and have run summits for hundreds of organization members in military, business, medical, and educational contexts, among others (Cooperrider & Sekerka, 2003).

Lind and Smith (2008) used the strengths-based approach of appreciative inquiry to build a bridge between discourse and practice in Canada. They describe how AI helped nurses and leaders of a local First Nations community collaboratively develop a new framework for community health nursing. As the nurses gained greater insights into traditional practices and the community's need to incorporate their culture into health care, community members developed a greater appreciation of the nurses' contribution to their well-being. The process produced mutual genuine respect for peoples' lived experiences. For the nurses, the questioning and deconstructing of long-held values, beliefs, and assumptions underlying health delivery services and relationships was critical to producing a partnership model of development and a transformative, appreciative health-promoting agenda.

Talley, Rushing, and Gee (2005) used Cowling's (2001) unitary appreciative inquiry process – based on the AI approach and Martha Rogers' theory of unitary human beings – to introduce RN-to-BSN students to an innovative way of working with a community. The students were asked to profile a small rural community. Prior to entering the community, the students were introduced to Cowling's unitary appreciative inquiry process and oriented according to the following steps (Talley, Rushing, & Gee, pp. 31-32):

- Check out your attitude about the community. Acknowledge any prejudices, fears, or concerns and put them out of your way.

- Practice noticing. Hear what people have to say, what they talk about, what they think about, and what they mean.

- Relax and allow the community to tell its story to you. Engage with the community.

- Feel yourself immersing in the community and connecting with the people who live there.

- Look at them with eyes of respect and a valuing approach. Be thankful for them and what they can share with you. Appreciate them and their way of life.

- Also, value your own intuition and your own ways of knowing.

- Find joy in the experience and keep it with you.

The students created a short film about the community and shared it with attendees at a conference. Feedback from audience members conveyed their sense that the film made them feel present in this small community with which they were unfamiliar. Credit was given to the unitary appreciative inquiry process (Cowling, 2001) for allowing the students to "be" in the community, to convey the essence of the community in a caring and respectful way. The community's strengths were appreciated and its system was respected – the only context in which concerns about health could be addressed. The students were innovative in their intervention.

As these examples show, for global service-learning to improve the health and well-being of different populations, it is imperative to view communities as resources for further development, rather than as problems to be solved. Often, participants in service-learning who hold a prescriptive approach to working with a host community become frustrated when met with resistance. It is confusing for them when the community does not seem to value what the service-learners are trying to do for them. Service-learners who appreciate diversity, can tolerate uncertainty, and possess a sense of humility are in the best position to have a rewarding experience.

Principles of Appreciative Inquiry

After a number of years of studying how people ask questions, Cooperrider and Srivastva (1987) posited that the most important lesson from appreciative inquiry is that people move in the direction of what they most seriously, frequently, and authentically ask questions about. Rather than assigning blame, appreciative inquiry reframes the questions toward success and creative opportunities (Preskill & Catsambas, 2006). This approach leads to collaboration and innovative exploration.

Cooperrider and Srivastva (1987) presented four guiding principles that should direct inquiry into the potential of organizational life. (1) Inquiry should begin with *appreciation*, meaning it should look for the best in the system under examination. (2) Inquiry should be *applicable*, meaning that the outcomes of the process should be meaningful to the community in which the inquiry takes place, and should be validated in action. (3) Inquiry should be *provocative*, meaning that it should generate knowledge, models, and images that are compelling to the community and that provoke people in the community to take action from an enlightened perspective. (4) Finally, inquiry should be *collaborative*, meaning that community representatives must be partners in the design and execution of the inquiry. These four principles form a foundation for openness and experimentation in the specifics of appreciative inquiry (Bushe & Kassam, 2005).

In the context of service-learning, the appreciative inquiry process could begin by asking host community members to share success stories about their experiences. Sharing stories builds a foundation by which positive relationships are developed and sustained, as the partners discover common grounds for understanding. During this process, bonds of trust in the partnership are likely to develop, and openness in communication is established.

The story-sharing phase of appreciative inquiry corresponds to the first stage in a four-step process developed by Cooperrider and Sekerka (2003): Discovery, Dream, Design, and Destiny, or the 4Ds. The 4Ds offer a means of organizing the process of change and creating questions. Participants should keep the four principles of inquiry in mind as they follow these four steps.

Following the first phase, *discovery* of their strengths, participants systematically move to step 2, the *dream*. During this phase, partners apply their strengths to a vision of an ideal future, sharing their hopes and goals. If all goes well, trust mounts and is sustained as the partners develop their vision, purpose, and strategic plan.

Step 3, *design*, is the phase that involves taking risks. This is the point where the details of a project are laid out. At this stage in the game, the service-learners and host community partners test provocative propositions that lead towards reinventing the community. The work builds on the first two steps and establishes very high levels of interpersonal and communal trust.

Finally, the opportunity to live the design and reach a *destiny* is realized in step 4, as the plans laid out in step 3 are brought to fruition. This step is about implementation of the plan, but not only that; it is about the transformation of paradigms (Cooperrider, Whitney & Stavros , 2003).

Living the experience of transformation based on appreciative inquiry with the host community creates sustainability, built on a firm foundation of mutual respect, trust, empathy, and understanding. The process is highly interactive and engaging; one might even call it infectious. In this, it resembles another model that puts systems theory and appreciative inquiry into practice: the World Café.

Systems Theory and Appreciative Inquiry in Practice: The World Café

The World Café is a set of principles and processes used to evoke collective intelligence and link it to effective action in pursuit of common aims (The World Cafe, n.d.). The idea of the World Café is to recreate the intimate, relaxed setting of a coffee-shop where participants can share their thoughts in small groups, allowing original and creative ideas to emerge. The World Café system has been adopted by a growing global community of groups, organizations, and networks. Many World Café participants and practitioners have found the technique to be effective in overcoming barriers, releasing collective wisdom, and promoting informed creative action.

Six principles of the World Café create an environment for discovery:

- Set the context

- Create a hospitable space

- Explore questions that matter

- Encourage everyone's contribution

- Connect diverse perspectives

- Listen together and notice patterns

- Share collective discoveries

The World Café technique can be used in specific settings to foster creative thinking among members of an organization or partners in a dialogue. As a broader system, the World Café can be thought of as a living network of conversations continually co-evolving with family, friends, colleagues, and community. The metaphor of the "World as Café" focuses on the invisible webs of dialogue and personal relationships that motivate learning, create shared purpose, and shape co-created life-affirming futures. The process aligns with appreciative inquiry's discovery phase. Rather than unfocused conversation in this discovery period, exploring questions that matter helps to shape the direction of the interaction. Questions in the direction of what people see as most serious to them, frequently pondered, and authentically viewed become the questions to explore.

In this regard, "explore questions that matter" is the most important of the six Café principles, the one that most determines whether the outcome of the process – in our case, designing and shaping a global service-learning initiative – will be meaningful and sustainable. Knowledge emerges in response to compelling questions that are relevant to the real-life concerns of the group. Powerful questions that "travel well" help generate collective energy, insights, and action as they move through the system. What makes a powerful question? Over time, World Café practitioners have distilled the experiences of hundreds of people to suggest the following: Questions should be simple and clear, thought-provoking, and focused, and should open new possibilities and invite deeper reflection. Depending on the project's timeframe and objectives, the "explore questions that matter" principle may be used to look at a single question or to develop a progressively deeper line of inquiry through several conversational rounds.

Summary

In this chapter, I have strived to explain how a theoretical framework incorporating systems theory and appreciative inquiry can strengthen global service-learning partnerships. A systems theory approach encourages a broad contextual understanding of the interacting relationships in a system prior to designing and evaluating interventions. An understanding of systems makes it easier to see how changes in one area might affect other areas and the system as a whole, and makes it more likely that a partnership will plan interventions with reasonably predictable outcomes. Appreciative inquiry offers a positive perspective that promotes learning from success and building capacity.

Participation in a global service-learning experience can lead to self-reflection and self-discovery, and to the acquisition of skills and values that undergird a broader appreciation of communities and the relationships between the community and the individual. General systems theory and appreciative inquiry together provide a model for a global service-learning approach that will help ensure long-term success for such endeavors, benefiting both vulnerable and marginalized communities and the students who serve them.

References

Bushe, G. R., & Kassam, A. F. (2005). When is appreciative inquiry transformational? A meta-case analysis. *The Journal of Applied Behavioral Science, 41*(2),161-181.

Cooperrider, D. L., & Godwin, L. N. (2010, August 10). Positive organization development: Innovation-inspired change in an economy and ecology of strengths. Retrieved from http://appreciativeinquiry.case.edu/intro/IPOD_draft_8-26-10.pdf.

Cooperrider, D., & Sekerka, L. E. (2003). Elevation of inquiry into the appreciable world: Toward a theory of positive organizational change. In K. Cameron, J. Dutton, and R. Quinn (Eds.), *Positive organizational scholarship* (pp. 225-240). San Francisco: Berrett-Kohler.

Cooperrider, D. L., & Srivastva, S. (1987). Appreciative inquiry in organizational life. In W. W. Pasmore (Ed.), *Research in organizational change and development. Vol. 1*, (pp. 129- 169), Greenwich: JAI Press.

Cowling, W. R. (2001). Unitary appreciative inquiry. *Advances in Nursing Science, 23*(4), 32-48..

de Savigny, D., & Adam, T. E. (2009). *Systems thinking for health systems strengthening.* Geneva: World Health Organization.

Lasker, R. D., & Weiss, E. S. (2002). *Maximizing the power of collaboration. Community-Campus Partnerships for Health (CCPH) Pre-Conference Workshop.* Miami: Center for the Advancement of Collaborative Strategies in Health, New York Academy of Medicine.

Lind, C., & Smith, D. (2008). Analyzing the state of community health nursing: Advancing from deficit to strengths-based practice using appreciative inquiry. *Advances In Nursing Science, 31*(1), 28-41.

Preskill, H., & Catsambas, T. T. (2006). *Reframing evaluation through appreciative inquiry.* Thousand Oaks, CA: Sage Publications, Inc.

Stanhope, M., & Lancaster, J. (2010). *Foundations of nursing in the community: Community-oriented practice* (3rd ed.). St Louis: Mosby.

Sword, W., Reutter, L., Meagher-Stewart, D., & Rideout, E. (2004). Baccalaureate nursing students' attitudes toward poverty: Implications for nursing curricular. *Journal of Nursing Education, 43*(1), 13-19.

Talley, B., Rushing, A., & Gee, R. M. (2005). Community assessment using Cowling's unitary appreciative inquiry: A beginning exploration. *Journal of Rogerian Nursing Science, 13*(1), 27–40.

The World Cafe. (n.d.). Cafe Principles in Action. Retrieved from http://www.theworldcafe.com/principles.html

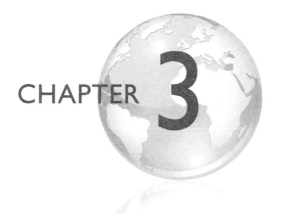

CHAPTER 3

Developing and Sustaining a Global Service-Learning
Program in Nursing: A Four-Step Approach

Tamara H. McKinnon
Gerard M. Fealy

Many programs in nursing include global service-learning (GSL) opportunities for students and experienced nurses. While these programs vary in focus and scope as well as in the characteristics of participants, GSL programs typically entail an immersion experience in a community at a geographical location removed from the participants' own community. This essential feature exemplifies nursing's commitment to educate and train its workforce in recognizing and responding to the health needs and challenges of global communities, including at-risk communities. GSL is therefore part of nursing's response to particular global challenges, such as the spread of communicable disease and the terrorist threat (Carlton, Ryan, Ali, & Kelsey, 2007).

This chapter offers a guide to program development in GSL in nursing. The four steps outlined are based on the authors' personal experiences, as well as a review of relevant literature.

Principles of Global Service-Learning

Community engagement is a core academic and scholarly activity (Holland & Gelmon, 1998) expressed in a range of activities, including community immersion and service-learning. Service-learning creates a dynamic partnership between communities and institutions of higher education, so that both the community and the institution benefit (Peterson & Schaffer, 1999). The relationship meets a particular community need and also affords program participants opportunities to develop their knowledge and skills in an experiential learning mode. GSL offers the learner a rich opportunity to actively participate in learning and service within the context of a unique culture and community. GSL also involves transformative learning, which places the learner more in the role of participant and less in the role of observer (Newman, 2008).

In the case of nursing students, service-learning contributes to the development of their role as nurses while fostering a sense of social responsibility and other capacities for good citizenship (Nokes, Nickitas, Keida, & Neville, 2005). Among these is cultural competence, including an understanding of the social and cultural contexts in which their nursing skills may be deployed in the future (Eyler, 2002). Culturally competent graduates are those who can, in Wehling's (2008) words, "address the paradigms of inequality and invisibility while allowing community partners to discover how to advocate for one another" (p. 293). However, for any single service-learning project to be ethical and sustainable, it should be with reference to the self-articulated needs of the community in receipt of the service and not imposed by the service provider. Projects that are faculty-initiated can be both difficult to start and difficult to maintain when compared with those based on invited opportunities (Memmott et al., 2010). Hence, a project or program is more likely to be sustained if the host community and the service provider develop a relationship built on mutual understanding and clear expectations and aimed at meeting needs of both partners (Immonen, Anderssen, & Lvova, 2008). A key outcome for a GSL program is that it leaves a host community in a better position, particularly with reference to self-advocacy and self-reliance.

Memmott et al. (2010) suggest essential features of program development that must be handled appropriately in order to build a sustainable program of international experiences for nursing students. These are: finding a fit within the mission of the university; working with the college and university operational structure; selecting faculty and students; developing the site; designing the course; and evaluating the program. These factors constitute the practical considerations of program development and require resources as well as commitment on the part of both faculty and students.

In this chapter, we offer four basic but essential steps for program development that address planning, method, relationship building, and program evaluation. The four steps are directed at prospective program leaders in GSL nursing programs. The steps will also be helpful in the design of observational and other study abroad programs.

Step One: Program Planning

Program planning involves asking and answering the "why," "where," "who," and "when" questions of program development. The initial impetus for program development may be a decision to take action based on a particular desire on the part of the program leader to engage in GSL with students. In other cases, it may be the sudden realization that an opportunity has arisen and the timing is right for action. Regardless of how one makes the decision to develop a GSL program in nursing, the initial planning steps are critical in the design of an effective and sustainable program.

Why: The rationale

At the outset, a prospective program leader must ask: what is my motivation in pursuing GSL program development? It is incumbent on the prospective leader to have a clear understanding of his or her own motivation in order to be successful in the leader role. A number of factors may motivate individual faculty members to pursue GSL program development. These include the failure of current curriculum models to meet the needs of nursing students who are likely to encounter diverse patients in a variety of clinical settings (Calvillo et al., 2009), and recognition of the potential in applied scholarship and community-based learning for enhancing community relations and the overall performance of the institution (Holland & Gelmon, 1998). Prospective GLS program leaders in nursing will certainly also recognize the potential impact that academic-community partnerships can have on the community partner. For underserved populations, point-of-living service delivery has the potential to make a difference in their lives, including having greater access to health care and much-needed resources, resolution of problems, and the potential for improving their health status (Lough, 1999). However, motivation that is based on a personal crusade may cloud the leader's judgments in planning.

Whatever the motivation, program development must be consistent with the mission, vision, and values of the leader's parent institution (Holland & Gelmon, 1998; Memmott et al., 2010), while also representing a "global vision for healthier communities" (Quigley, Sayers, & Hanson, 1998, p.127). Effective GLS programs are those that provide participants with opportunities to develop competencies related to culture, collaboration, communication, and research, and afford the host community opportunities to build its capacity for self-development (Frank, 2008). A key outcome is the development of culturally competent graduates who can address community problems, such as health inequalities, and who can help communities to be self-advocates (Wehling, 2008).

Where: The host/partner community

The establishment of a relationship with the host community can originate in a number of ways. The program leader may have an existing connection with members of a community, and the concept of a collaborative endeavor emanates from that relationship. Alternately, the leader may initiate contact with a community because its demographics, health issues, or other factors are consistent with a desired program focus. The initial connection may be made with an international professional group, such as the International Council of Nursing or Sigma Theta Tau International. Regardless of how the relationship with a partner community originates, it is imperative that the program leader identify community leaders and other stakeholders in the host community, in order to set the stage for a sustainable collaborative relationship.

The partner community may have already participated in one or more GSL initiatives, or it may be new to such activities. Since participant welfare is a key concern, when selecting a partner that is new, consideration should be given to the particular circumstances of the host country in which the partner is located, including the host country's political stability and the stability of its health system (Memmott et al., 2010). Other practical issues to be considered in the planning phase include possible language barriers, and participants' health and safety, such as the need for participant inoculations or special clothing and footwear.

When assessing the host community and its needs, the GSL program leader has a range of assessment methods at her/his disposal, including a comprehensive community assessment, a literature review, and one-to-one discussions with liaisons and community leaders. At the outset, it is necessary to be clear about what constitutes a community but at the same time to recognize that it may not always be possible or even necessary to develop a single definition of what the community is (Holland & Gelmon, 1998). Rather, it is the context in which the institution and community interact and the nature of shared effort that gives rise to the definition, and also to the effective institution-community partnership (Holland & Gelmon). As Holland and Gelmon (p. 107) write: "We describe effective partnerships as knowledge-based collaborations in which all partners have things to teach each other, things to learn from each other, and things they will learn together [and] … build the capacity of each partner to accomplish its own mission while also working together." Program planners have a responsibility to ensure that programs have a focus on community empowerment, thereby avoiding the development of dependent relationships (Walsh, 2004).

Who: Home institution, partner community, and program participants

It is important for GSL program leaders to identify the partners in any new endeavor. Programs will be successful only when all participants are included in the planning. Broadly, GSL partners are the program leader(s), the home institution, the host community, and the participants.

Partner clarification requires the leader to have a clear understanding of the mission and role of his/her own institution. For example, contractual arrangements, such as memoranda of understanding, may name the entire home institution, the school, or simply the leader's own division in a nursing school or health care organization. The name of the leader and any named collaborator or associate leader and the names of individual faculty, clinical nurses, and administrators should be recorded and their respective roles in the program should be clearly delineated. Successful community engagement requires the identification and support of faculty leaders and mentors who will have the staying power to sustain the partnership and its related activities over time, and who will integrate community engagement into their overall scholarly agenda (Holland & Gelmon, 1998).

The host community partner must also be clearly identified, and the rationale for selecting a particular host community should be explicit. At a contractual level, the host community might be a national or state government, a local municipal authority, or a local institution, such as a hospital, school, or community health facility. A named contact person in the host community should be identified at an early stage in the process and this person should be readily contactable. The relationship between the leader and the contact person is critical and should be one that is built on mutual respect from the outset. Open communications must be initiated and there should be regular contacts during the planning phase, with a subsidiary function of offering mutual support to the individuals involved.

The criteria for selecting program participants should be developed early, and clearly communicated to all prospective participants and to all others concerned. The first step is to determine the population from which candidates may be drawn. While much of the literature focuses on nursing students as GSL participants, experienced nurses have much to gain from and much to contribute to a GSL program.

Referring to the selection of students for study abroad programs, Memmott et al. (2010) stress the importance of selecting participants who have the attributes to adapt to new and challenging situations, including "adequate nursing knowledge and skills, interpersonal skills, cultural sensitivity, maturity, and flexibility" (p. 301). Moreover, the participants are ambassadors for nursing, their sponsoring school, their university, and their country (Memmott et al., 2010). How students respond to their experience and how they communicate their experience to prospective future participants can influence how the program is perceived and can ultimately influence its sustainability.

Once participants are selected, their names should be recorded. Program participants then need to be involved in aspects of the planning that directly or indirectly affect them and their future experiences on the program.

When: Timing

The timing of the decision to initiate a GLS program is also important. It is essential to allow sufficient time for program planning and development; experience suggests that this takes up to a year or more. Questions around timing concern the readiness of the home institution and/or the host community to participate. Readiness refers to issues affecting administrative and planning arrangements, such as travel, climate, and so forth, but also to psychological readiness on the part of individuals in either the home institution or the host community. If either partner is not ready, there is a greater risk of failure.

Too often prospective program leaders begin planning without having completed the requisite initial assessments. Equally, they may be eager to move forward with a program and embark on program development in the late planning stage. Thus, they may make logistical decisions without the benefit of comprehensive assessment and clarification of the program's focus or the host's capacity to fully participate in the program. This frequently leads to frustration on the part of the leader, the partner community, and participants when it becomes apparent that the program was not designed with consideration of the needs and abilities of all parties in mind. Relevant learning objectives and program activities must be determined, based on comprehensive assessment of the community partner, home institution, and program participants.

Begin the process of GSL program development by asking the "why," "where," "who," and "when" questions. During this process, remember to address the potential ethical

Table 3-1. Sources and Timing of Evaluative Data

ollect information from... hen:	Participants	Host/partner community	Home institution	Program leader
e-program				
ost-program				
months post-program				

In the evaluation process, it is essential that the effects of GSL programs on host mmunities be carefully examined. Partner communities often report that they appreciate e focused work provided by GSL team members, but some have expressed concerns er inconsistency in approach and a lack of focus on strength-based interventions ommunity-Campus Partnerships for Health [CCPH], 2003). Evaluation topics related to st communities may include whether the program has enhanced community capacity, ether it has led to a long-term collaboration, and whether it has resulted in joint search and publications. Joint research and publications are a tangible expression of a eaningful and effective partnership.

Few studies have reported on how GSL programs have affected program leaders or eir institutions. This paucity of evidence presents opportunities to explore topics such the integration of a long-term collaborative program into the institutional mission and sion; and program outcomes from the perspective of the program leader.

Conclusion

e have proposed a four-step guide to effective and sustainable global service-learning rogram development, based on the literature and our own experiences developing GSL ograms. In this guide, we address the key stages of planning, method, relationship uilding, and program evaluation. Step one involves exploration related to the questions "why," "where," "who," and "when." Step two concerns the "what" and "how" of rogram development. Step three focuses on relationships between stakeholders, such as e program leader, home institution, program participants, and the host community. Step ur deals with evaluation of the program and moving toward the future, with a focus on ctions to promote sustainability.

A successful GSL project offers benefits for all parties concerned. For program

issues that might arise in entering a new community to provide a service, and ensure that ethical concerns are integrated into each stage of planning.

A prospective GLS program leader needs to be clear as to the precise focus of the program that is to be developed. Will the program be focused on service, on education, or a combination of the two? This gives rise to the "what" and "how" questions, the question of method.

Step Two: Method

GSL is one of a number of approaches to developing student learning. Other similar and related program types include study abroad programs and international immersion learning experiences. Frank (2008) provides examples of collaborative academic-service partnerships, including service programs, educational programs, and service-learning programs. Each program type has its own particular aims.

An international immersion experience combined with a service-learning methodology can provide an excellent opportunity for students to develop cultural competence, and can also enable nursing faculty to meet the challenge of educating nurses who are prepared to deliver quality care in the multicultural context.

With this in mind, step two addresses the "what" and "how" questions of GSL program development. Here, we cover only the "what". Other chapters in this volume describe the "how" in rich detail, particularly Chapters 4 and 5.

What and how: Clarify the program's vision and parameters

Once an assessment is complete, determine if the home institution, partner community, and program participants are in agreement regarding their goals and objectives. The focus of the program must be based on mutual aims and aspirations, with the interests and capacities of the host/partner community taking precedence. It is only when a host community's own resources and strengths are identified and used that the partnership will be sustainable, and the community will move closer to self-sufficiency (Holland & Gelmon, 1998).

Clarifying the program's vision involves developing a mission statement that lays out the goals and objectives for the program. On the basis that a service-learning program is aimed at attempting to help a community grow, the main tenets of appreciative inquiry can apply in the operation of the program. As a method of organizational or community development and as a practice-oriented activity, appreciative inquiry is a "cooperative co-evolutionary" process that seeks to establish the best in a community and its people and promotes community change by marshalling its untapped resources for transformation and growth (Cooperrider & Whitney, 2005). The community's positive core of assets, strengths and resources, including its people, is the basis for building, or co-creating, the community and its capacity for self-development into the future. The steps in the process of appreciative inquiry include valuing the community's own strengths, envisioning what might be, and dialoguing what ought to be (Cooperrider & Whitney, 2005).

At a practical level, when setting out the operation of the program, it is essential to identify roles and responsibilities along with expected outcomes for each partner. For example, while participants are acting in the role of learner, their learning is transformative and experiential, and as active participants in the community in which they are providing a service, they are required to take responsibility for key tasks and functions.

Step Three: Building Relationships

Successful implementation of steps one and two will increase the likelihood of effective on-site engagement among all partners. Programs are more likely to function smoothly if there is careful and deliberate planning, based on a mutually agreed upon realistic schedule that includes time for project work, team meetings, reflective activities, and rest.

Beginning each program with an intensive on-site orientation maximizes involvement by partner community leaders and representatives and is a means of making participants feel more comfortable in their new surroundings. Relevant topics for initial orientation sessions include local history, culture, government and politics, and health care delivery, with a particular focus on nursing. Such orientation sessions present an opportunity for the leader and participants to review the program goals and related activities, and importantly, enable the development of rapport and team building.

Program participants who are well prepared for the global experience are equipped to move quickly into implementation of service activities. Commencing work on the community project as soon as possible after arrival in the host community enables participant engagement, creates service momentum, and provides participants with a sense of purpose. It also helps to clarify the role of participants within the project team. Since participants can expect to experience a certain degree of homesickness and role confusion (Lee, 2004), it is important to integrate time for group discussions and individual time with the leader, in order to allow participants to process issues that may arise.

Regularly scheduled collaborative group meetings provide community stakeholders with the opportunity to present their perspective on progress toward the attainment of service goals. Leaders from the host community should be given opportunities to review project status, project costs, and the effectiveness of collaborative endeavors. By making sure all stakeholders have a chance to take stock and can provide input into decisions

about altering community activities, the likelihood is increased that effec[tive] relationships will develop.

While the program leader has built up a range of institutional supp[ort] in the course of planning the project, once embedded in the host comm[unity] may have to operate relatively autonomously in facilitating the progra[m] can feel threatening to the leader. The authors' experiences suggest t[hat] characteristics will serve program leaders well during this formative and experience. An ability to be focused, flexible, curious, and enthusiastic take new challenges in stride without feeling overwhelmed.

Once community service activities become established, they can be c sustained by paying close attention to participant engagement and comm with the focus on enabling the community to contribute to the progra strengths. This paves the way for successful planning for subsequent g for continuation of the service project with input from community memb activities such as establishing a schedule related to community activit based progress toward self-sufficiency being a critical step prior to projec

Step Four: Program Evaluation

The final step of GSL program development involves determining the program from the perspective of all partners, utilizing agreed-upon qua measurement tools. In evaluating the program, success should be de perspective of the community, the participants, and the institution; lik outcomes should be measured with reference to community, participant, pre-program objectives (Holland & Gelmon, 1998). For example, from of program participants, evaluations could be designed to measure their self-awareness, cultural competence, civic engagement, teamwork, and c skills. Long-term follow-up can show how participants integrate knowle gained from their service-learning experience into their careers as profe (Evanson & Zust, 2006; Lee, 2004).

Assessment methodologies for program evaluation may include pre- for participants, questionnaires, personal conversations with community participants, and review of participant journals and blogs. At a minim and summative evaluation can be based on information obtained prior to immediately following the program, and at a point in time removed completion (see Table 3-1).

participants, immersion in another community beyond their immediate borders provides a unique opportunity to learn about another culture, its customs, environment, and particular health needs, thereby enhancing the participant's knowledge, nursing skills and cultural competence. For the served community, a particular community need is addressed, and the community is given the opportunity to become healthier and to develop greater self-reliance. For program planners, the experience offers the satisfaction of contributing to a project with direct and tangible benefits for students, communities and their own professional and personal development. The current chapter offers a roadmap that, we hope, will help program leaders as they embark on the difficult, sometimes frightening process of developing these important and valuable programs.

References

Calvillo, E., Clark, L., Ballantyne, J. E., Pacquiao, D., Purnell, L. D., & Villarruel, A. M. (2009). Cultural competency in baccalaureate nursing education. *Journal of Transcultural Nursing, 20*(2), 137–145.

Carlton, K., Ryan, M., Ali, N., & Kelsey, B. (2007). Integration of global health concepts in nursing curricula: A national study. *Nursing Education Perspectives, 28*(3), 124–129.

Community-Campus Partnerships for Health. (2003). Service-learning in the health professions: Advancing educational innovations for improved student learning and community health. *CCPH 7th Annual Introductory Service-Learning Institute Proceedings,* Leavenworth, WA. Available at: http://www.ccph (Retrieved December 15, 2010).

Cooperrider, D. L., & Whitney, D. (2005). *Appreciative inquiry: A positive revolution in change*. San Francisco: Barrett-Koehler.

Evanson, R., & Zust, B. (2006). 'Bittersweet knowledge': The long-term effects of an international experience. *Journal of Nursing Education, 45*(10), 412–419.

Eyler, J. (2002). Reflecting on service: Helping nursing students get the most from service-learning. *Journal of Nursing Education 4*(10), 453–456.

Frank, B. (2008). Enhancing nursing education through effective academic-service partnerships. *Annual Review of Nursing Education, 6,* 625–643.

Holland, B., & Gelmon, S. B. (1998). The state of the 'engaged campus': What we have learned about building and sustaining university-community partnerships. *American Association of Higher Education Bulletin, 51*(2), 3–6.

Immonen, I., Anderssen, N., & Lvova, M. (2008). Project work across borders in the arctic Barents region: Practical challenges for project members. *Nurse Education Today, 28,* 841–848.

Lee, N. J. (2004). The impact of international experience on student nurses' personal and professional development. *International Nursing Review, 51*(2), 113–122.

Lough, M. A. (1999). An academic-community partnership: A model of service and education. *Journal of Community Health Nursing, 16*(3), 137–149.

Memmott, R. J., Coverston, C. R., Hcisc, B. A., Williams, M., Maughan, C. D., Kohl, J., & Palmer, S. (2010). Practical considerations in establishing sustainable international nursing experiences. *Nursing Education Perspectives, 31*(5), 298–302.

Newman, M. (2008). *Transforming presence: The difference that nursing makes.* Philadelphia: FA Davis Company.

Nokes, K. M., Nickitas, D. M., Keida, R., & Neville, S. (2005). Does service-learning increase cultural competency, critical thinking, and civic engagement? *Journal of Nursing Education, 44*(2), 65–70.

Peterson, S., & Schaffer, M. (1999). Service learning: A strategy to develop group collaboration and research skills. *Journal of Nursing Education, 38*(5), 208–214.

Quigley, E., Sayers, B., & Hanson, R. (1998). Service-learning lessons from the chambered nautilus. In J. Norbeck, C. Connolly, & J. Koerner (Eds.), *Caring and community concepts and models for service-learning in nursing* (pp.119-127). San Francisco, CA: American Association for Higher Education.

Walsh, D. S. (2004). A framework for short-term humanitarian health care projects. *International Nursing Review, 51*, 23–26.

Wehling, S. (2008). Cross-cultural competency through service-learning. *Journal of Community Practice, 16*(3), 293–315.

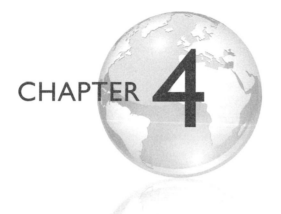

CHAPTER 4

Home Institution Responsibilities and Best Practices

Marilyn Blakenship Lotas

The development of a global service-learning (GSL) program is a major undertaking for any school of nursing, combining the challenges of creating a study abroad program with the added complexity of the service-learning model itself. It requires a significant commitment of administrative leadership, faculty time, and institutional resources for both planning and implementation of a program, and an equal commitment to maintaining it once it has been established.

The decision to integrate a GSL experience into the educational process of a nursing program is grounded in an awareness of the extraordinary transformations in information, communication, health, and health services occurring throughout our global community; in recognition that over the coming decades nurses must be prepared to practice in an increasingly culturally diverse world; and in a commitment to serve in the communities where we learn. A study abroad experience can lead to a better understanding of another culture. A global service-learning experience can add a deeper level of engagement, empathy with that culture, and greater insight into how the dynamics of that culture impact the health of its members.

To be optimally successful, a global service-learning program will not be a single isolated event in a nursing program. It should be the culmination of a series of educational experiences designed to provide the student with, minimally,

- an understanding of the service-learning model;
- a basic understanding of the concepts of culture, health, and health care and their interactions;
- a model for completing a community assessment and identifying factors contributing to or impeding the health care of that community; and
- a systematic approach to the development of a community-based project.

(The Dreyfus Health Foundation's Problem Solving for Better Health model [http://www.dhfglobal.org/who/psbhi.html] is an example of a model that can be successfully taught to and used by undergraduate students in the development of community-based health projects.)

Regardless of the type or length of the GSL experience, whether it meets a curriculum requirement or is an enrichment opportunity, its value to the individual student and to the nursing program will be enhanced to the degree that the experience is seen as contributing directly to the student's overall nursing education.

Global service-learning programs come in many sizes and shapes, each bringing its own set of challenges and concerns. Each model must address in some way multiple factors, including the conceptualization of the experience itself; the development of the partnership with the host site; the selection, preparation and advisement of students;

the supervision of the experience; and the evaluation of outcomes. Initially, two aspects are of particular importance in identifying the issues that need to be addressed in the development of a GSL experience: 1) is the program short (e.g., a few weeks) or long (a semester or academic year), and 2) is the program faculty-led, or will the students be at the site without direct supervision from the home institution? Each of these aspects will be discussed in terms of best practices for preplanning and site development; student selection, advisement and preparation; student project development and oversight; supervision; post-experience debriefing; and outcome evaluation.

Throughout this chapter, I will reference the "Standards of Good Practice for Education Abroad" developed by the Forum on Education Abroad (4th edition, 2011), available at http://www.forumea.org/standards-standards.cfm. Planners should refer to these Standards as they undertake each stage in GSL program development.

Preplanning and Development

The preplanning phase involves asking and answering questions, including what educational issues or goals are to be addressed by the experience; why it is important in terms of the mission and philosophy of the overall program; and how a global service-learning experience will contribute to the overall goals of the program. In addition, the program leader will want to consider what infrastructure is in place in the home institution to support a GSL project. Each of these questions will begin to inform the planning process. (Standards of Good Practice, 2011: Standards 1 and 7.)

Internal School of Nursing Issues

The initial step in the planning process is to begin to describe the purpose and outcomes of the proposed experience and its relationship to the program curriculum. Is it to be an "additive" experience that contributes to the student's educational experience but is not part of the required curriculum, or is it to be an integral curriculum component fulfilling a graduation requirement? These questions correspond to the two issues raised above as central to the shaping of a GSL experience: Will the program be short or long, and will it be led by faculty members from the home institution? Typically, shorter-term experiences do not comprise an integral part of the curriculum; these experiences tend to be faculty-led. A program that replaces a required course will most often be longer (a semester or more) and will not require the presence of home-institution faculty. Although there are unique issues for each type of experience, both types must have clear educational objectives and planning for instruction, supervision and oversight, and evaluation. (Standards of Good Practice, 2011: Standard 3.)

Short-term experiences can be extremely valuable and provide a great deal of flexibility as to the type of experience, activities involved, length of the experience, academic credit given, and evaluation methods. These experiences are most commonly one to three weeks in length and, as noted above, are faculty-led. Most global service-learning experiences will fall into this category. The distinguishing factor is that, while academic credit is given, most often the course will not replace a required nursing course. Preplanning focuses on the development of clear educational objectives, consideration of the type of activities and sites that will meet those objectives, and how oversight and program evaluation will be implemented. Experiences may at times evolve from an opportunity or site that becomes available, followed by consideration of what kinds of experiences might be developed for that site. However, most successful experiences will be initiated after thoughtful preplanning, involving a clear sense of the outcomes to be achieved and the kind of site that will best support meeting these outcomes.

The second type of experience, one that is integral to the required curriculum, requires additional consideration. These experiences are typically longer in duration, lasting one or two semesters. In addition to developing the educational objectives, activities, required products and plans for oversight and evaluation of the experience, the program leader needs to make decisions about what course or courses will "house" the experience, how it will meet course objectives, and how it will contribute to the overall curriculum. It is also important in this preplanning phase to explore issues related to having the courses included on the student's transcript and ensuring that the course will meet relevant graduation requirements. Course activities and supervision arrangements must meet the requirements of the State Board of Nursing for nursing curricula, and activities must be within the scope of practice for a student nurse in the home state. (Standards of Good Practice, 2011: Standard 3.)

Broader Institutional Issues

For both types of programs, a second area of consideration that must be addressed is the home institution's mission and values related to study abroad. These are likely to include rules and regulations with specifications for inter-institutional contracts and required standards for study abroad programs. Specifications and standards may cover, for example: the academic merit of the experience; requirements for oversight and evaluation; documentation of institutional liability insurance; financial aid issues; legal disclaimers or indemnification of the home institution against legal claims; requirements for health and liability insurance; and, policies related to parental permission.

Policies related to student selection, advisement and preparation may also be in place. Other issues defined by the home institution will include who is responsible for financial commitments related to the program, and whether those expenses can be covered by financial aid. (Standards of Good Practice, 2011: Standard 6.)

Preplanning and Development of a Selected Site

Site Selection

When the program leader has identified the kind of experience desired, its length, and its relationship to the required curriculum, and has reviewed the home institution's study abroad requirements, it is time to identify the host site. Assuming that all GSL experiences give students an opportunity to work within a service-learning model and within a different culture, different program purposes will suggest different kinds of host sites. For instance, the program might be designed chiefly around the goal of fostering in students a sense of civic responsibility while providing health education and health care to an underserved population. It might be aimed at exposing students to a different kind of health care system, allowing them to compare health care delivery and outcomes in (for instance) a nationalized system versus the U.S. private-insurance system. The goal might be to increase students' cultural competence through immersion in a different culture. Or it might be to help students gain facility in another language in order to engage more effectively in the delivery of care.

A careful review of the purposes of the experience will help in identifying the general category or kind of site that would be appropriate, and in determining what level of engagement students will need. For instance, will the students be providing direct care to individuals, or will they engage chiefly in observation and other more general activities? In this regard, it is important to understand the host institution's policies regarding student activities, including policies related to direct patient involvement. It is equally important to impress upon everyone involved that the home institution's students may not exceed the standards and scope of student practice in the home institution, regardless of the policies existing in the host institution.

Site selection entails compiling a thoughtful inventory of potential sites, with consideration to where an individual program director or the home institution has established relationships to facilitate initial contacts; whether there is a language barrier and, if so, how will that be addressed; and what kind of host institution would most appropriately and effectively support the desired experience. For a short-term, faculty-led experience, host institutions could be clinics, hospitals, universities/schools, or other entities where health care is provided. For a semester-long or longer experience where home institution faculty will not be present at all times, there are distinct advantages in working with a school of nursing as the host institution. Schools of nursing will already have resources and protocols in place to address issues of safe and adequate student housing, student supervision, and student health and safety. These resources can potentially be engaged in support of visiting students. In addition, having the students enrolled in host school of nursing and/or university courses makes them eligible for many of the additional resources available for local students.

Negotiation with the Host Site

After identifying a potential site, initial contact can be made. Information provided at this time should include an overview of the service-learning model, a preliminary description of the proposed experience, and a course syllabus if one is available. It is important in the first contact to determine who in the potential site has the authority to negotiate and approve a contractual agreement and who in the home institution needs to "buy in" for the experience to succeed. At that point strategies can be developed to introduce the proposed experience to all involved constituencies. To do this will likely require a site visit and possibly presentations to the faculty and/or staff of the home institution. The endpoint of this first phase of the negotiation should be an informal agreement from both parties to proceed with planning the experience, along with a clear understanding and agreement on both sides regarding the project's educational and service objectives. At that point, the negotiations can move to the development of a formal interagency contract.

It must be emphasized that a primary consideration in site selection is the site's overall sense of safety. While this is important for all student experiences, it is particularly critical for experiences where no home institution faculty will be on-site. Any institution establishing this kind of experience must not only carefully evaluate the safety of the site initially, but must also be prepared to act immediately if a risk to student safety occurs.

Contract Negotiation

The elements of the contract governing the program will vary considerably from institution to institution based on the nature of the experience being planned and the cultures of both institutions. Minimally, the contract will specify the range of issues that are covered by the agreement, and the responsibility of both the home and host institutions for necessary resources, oversight, safety, supervision, and evaluation of the student experience. Agreements will also specify student responsibilities, such as acquiring all necessary immunizations, liability insurance, financial resources, and documentation of previous clinical experiences. Contracts must also specify the necessary qualifications for supervising faculty or preceptors, whether provided by the home institution or the host. Most institutions will have required language describing liability, indemnification, and risk management requirements.

In general, key issues that may be addressed in the contractual agreement include:

- **Student housing.** The contract may specify who is responsible for identifying appropriate housing for the students and for faculty if present, and who bears the financial responsibility for housing expenses.

- **Student supervision.** The contract should specify the standards for student supervision set by the State Board of Nursing governing the home institution, and establish that supervision at the host institution must meet the same standards as supervision at the home institution. If students are to be supervised by persons not licensed in the state of the home university, supervisors provided by the host institution should have preparation equivalent to nurses who would be qualified to provide student supervision in the home institution's jurisdiction. Both supervising personnel and students must be clear that the standards and scope of practice for nursing students in other jurisdictions are not different or lower than the standards in force in the home institution.

- **Health and safety issues.** The contract should specify standards governing the health and safety of students while they are engaged in a study abroad experience, including required immunizations, and health and liability insurance.

Preliminary Development of Guidelines for Student Projects

While final development of specific projects is likely to wait until the experience is under way and the students are on-site, preliminary discussions and the development of broad guidelines should begin during the initial negotiation with the host site. The home institution faculty should provide the timeline, identify the resources the student(s) will bring – including time, financial resources, and the skills or capacity of the participants – and provide some examples of projects previously completed in other settings. Some ideas of needs that potential projects could address on-site should be elicited from representatives of the host institution. In some situations, the representatives of the home and host institutions may identify the project during this initial negotiation. In others, final decisions are made with input from the selected students. Early in the preliminary discussions a decision should be made about whether Institutional Review Board (IRB) approval will be sought for potential projects, since in a short-term experience it may be impossible to gain IRB approval if the application is made after the experience has begun. The outcome of this negotiation should be clearly defined and mutually agreed upon project guidelines for the proposed experience and the procedure to be used to define specific projects.

Marketing, Student Selection, and Pre-Departure Preparation

Marketing

With the program planning complete, the host institution identified, and a completely executed contract in place, the marketing of the experience can begin. The marketing information should include: descriptions of the physical site and the host institution; an overview of the planned experiences; a description of who will be leading or supervising the program, whether a home institution faculty member or someone at the host institution; a description of the housing to be provided; and a statement of expenses for the experience. This last may be either a comprehensive set cost for the experience or an estimate of the costs, including travel expenses, housing, and meal costs. The student's financial commitment must be explicitly stated, along with a description of any expenses to be covered by the home institution. It is helpful to provide pictures of the site and, if possible, some of the people the students will meet and specific agencies or sites where activities will occur. In addition, the marketing information should explicitly describe the student selection process and preparation experiences required, with any student eligibility requirements or exclusion criteria clearly stated.

The marketing materials should also include any disclaimers related to the project. Examples include a statement that the faculty reserve the right to cancel a program if circumstances warrant, or the conditions under which fees will or will not be reimbursed. For clarification, examples of events that have necessitated program cancellation in the past may be given. These can include, for example, natural disasters such as a major earthquake, or a change in the host country's political climate. (Standards of Good Practice, 2011: Standard 5.)

Student Selection

Student selection issues will vary somewhat depending on the type of GSL program that has been developed, and will be particularly important for those experiences where no faculty from the home institution will be present. Prior to developing a student selection plan, faculty should consider the nature of the site and experience and determine what qualities are important for students who will be taking part. If a language other than English is spoken at the site, it is important to determine the level of proficiency in that language the student may need. Students going to Chile to attend classes and work in community clinics need at least conversational Spanish. Students going to Denmark will find that most Danes speak and understand English and fluency in Danish is not necessary. If a home institution faculty member will not be on-site with the students, it may be important to consider the students' dependability, maturity, and ability to work both independently and with a group. In any global service-learning experience the potential for unanticipated change is high, and so the students should have tolerance for ambiguity and openness to new experiences.

Once the necessary or preferred qualities are identified, the components of the selection process can be developed to assess those qualities. It should be emphasized that from the beginning, it is helpful to have more than one faculty member involved both in identifying criteria for selection and in evaluating individual applicants.

Academic achievement is commonly used as a selection criterion, with a grade point average of 3.0 being the usual standard for all study abroad experiences. Faculty letters of recommendation are helpful in identifying strong clinical performance (if the student will be giving direct care) and in assessing qualities such as dependability and maturity. Student application essays can be useful in determining motivation and understanding about the nature and purpose of the experience. Finally, personal interviews with the student will add another dimension to the evaluation and selection process.

One important component of the selection interview is giving applicants insight into some of the challenges they may confront at the site. For many students this program will be their first experience of being in a minority group, being in an environment where they don't understand the language, or being in a culture whose values and belief structure are very different from their own. Making this explicit in the interview may give the interviewer a sense of how well students will be able to cope with these experiences and whether they have had similar experiences in the past. At the same time, the interview process may give students the opportunity to anticipate and, to some degree, prepare for the kinds of experiences they may encounter. (Standards of Good Practice, 2011: Standard 5.)

Student Pre-Departure Preparation

Once students have been selected for the experience, the importance of advising and preparing them prior to the experience cannot be overemphasized. Basic issues include initiating the application processes for visas, housing, and admission to the host institution if appropriate. In addition, the home university may have application requirements for any study abroad program, including a school of nursing GSL project. Other issues include the establishment of academic goals and expectations; introduction to the culture and history of the host institution; and health and safety issues.

Academic goals and expectations. The establishment of academic goals and expectations is a continuation of the process begun with marketing and continued through the selection process. The marketing materials should include a broad statement of the goals and expectations for the project. The selection process should include an exploration of how the student understands these goals and expectations, and an evaluation of whether the student's personal goals are congruent with those of the program. During the pre-departure preparation, the discussion of goals and expectations should become more individual and explicit. The focus should be on identifying specific activities related to what the student hopes to accomplish, including required products such as reports, reflections, or presentations, as well as a specific discussion of the student evaluation process.

Culture and history. Introduction to the culture and history of the host community is an essential and potentially challenging part of the student preparation process. A basic understanding of the history and culture of the site should be required for all students, with explicit requirements for achieving that. The objective is not for the student to achieve any level of expertise about the culture of the site, but to become sensitized to important issues. Some strategies that can be useful are: review of materials from the host institution; reference lists related to the history and culture of the site; conference calls with host site representatives; social media connections with students in the host institution; intensive seminars taught at either the home or host institution; and information sessions led by people familiar with the site.

If it has not occurred previously, it is important during this pre-departure preparation to openly discuss some of the issues that may be confronted during the experience. As mentioned above, discussion about the experience of being in a minority is particularly important when the experience is not faculty-led, and particularly when the students will be working in pairs or small groups. Students who will be in a setting where they don't speak or understand the language may need to anticipate how that may feel. It may also be important to talk about the culture shock students may face when, for example, they are exposed to an area of extreme poverty for the first time. No amount of discussion will completely prepare students for the experiences they will encounter. However, discussions prior to departing can help the student in anticipate such experiences and consider how they might respond.

Health and safety. Concerns related to health and safety must be discussed with all students. While many issues may seem obvious to faculty experienced in travel, it is not safe to assume that less experienced students are equally aware. Basic health issues include ensuring that students have the appropriate immunizations and health insurance coverage. All students should be advised to visit a travel clinic or its equivalent to ensure that all immunizations are up to date, including any additional immunizations needed for a specific site. Students should be advised to contact their current health insurance provider to determine how coverage can be continued and utilized while abroad. In addition, travel insurance with an evacuation clause should be considered.

Students should be apprised of any infectious diseases that are particularly prevalent in the host environment, and instructed to talk with their health care provider about whether they are at heightened risk from such diseases. Management of prescription drugs should be discussed, as well as suggestions for supplies such as hand sanitizer or over-the-counter medications. In addition, students should be advised of food and water safety issues in the host country and any precautions they should take.

Basic safety concerns should be discussed. These include how to safely get money changed in the host environment, and precautions specific to the site, such as where it is safe to walk and standards for appropriate dress. Students should be reminded to walk in groups or pairs in unfamiliar areas. In this regard, it is helpful to arrange for a local "buddy" to help with the early orientation to the site.

The importance of following all laws of the host country should be emphasized. Many students erroneously believe that as American citizens, they are exempt from many local laws or that the U.S. government will intervene if they are accused of any violation.

Finally, there should be a review of all emergency procedures: who should be called in an emergency, how emergency health care is to be managed, and who can make health care decisions for a student if necessary. Particularly where a home institution faculty member is not present on-site, all students should have a mobile telephone that is functional on-site by which they both can be reached in an emergency and can call home. Arrangements may be made with their regular service provider, or they can obtain a local prepaid telephone in the host country. If no home institution faculty member is on-site during the experience, students should have an emergency number at the home institution that can be called round the clock, as well as an identified person on-site who will be available for emergencies. (Standards of Good Practice, 2011: Standard 8.)

Final Identification of Projects

The identification of a mutually agreed upon project that provides both value to the host site and a substantive learning experience for the student is central to the global service-learning model. It represents a major component of the work to be done within the experience, although it may or may not constitute the total work commitment on the part of the student.

Collaboration and Negotiation

As previously discussed, the project can be identified during the early negotiation process between representatives of the home and host institutions. This is often most practical when the length of the experience is short and students need to be able to start their activity immediately. However, where possible, the student's participation in the development of a project can be a valuable part of the learning experience. The process provides the student with practice in defining the scope of a project to fit the time and resources available, and in collaborating with host institution representatives to determine the specific parameters of a project. However, even though the student may actively negotiate the project with the host institution, if this project must meet specific educational goals for either a course requirement or a graduation requirement, the home institution faculty must retain final authority for approval.

Relevance, Complexity, and Scope

Collaboration around the development of a project can be facilitated by ensuring that clear guidelines are provided to the host institution or developed in the preliminary contract negotiation. The project needs to be both relevant, and appropriate in complexity and scope. The relevance of the final project is determined by both its service value to the host institution and its congruence with the learning objectives of the course or curriculum of which it is a part. For example, organizing a filing system might be of high value to the host but may not meet a learning objective for the experience. However, if such a project is framed as the development of a patient information system, it might meet the relevance criterion for both host and home institutions. The complexity and scope of a project must be weighed in terms of the student's level of professional development, the time available to complete the project, the resources available for the project, and whether it is to be a group or an individual project. The home institution faculty leader holds primary responsibility for ensuring that the final project agreed upon is relevant and appropriate in complexity and scope.

Project Oversight: Host vs. Home Institution

Responsibility for oversight of the project varies depending on the structure of the experience. When the experience is faculty-led, the responsibility for the students' work rests primarily with the faculty leader, while the host institution maintains primary responsible for their site resources, policies and procedures, and client population. At times an overlap in responsibilities occurs as students interface with the host institution's facility, clients, and procedures, and the host institution's personnel may provide some direct oversight of the students' work. However, the primary responsibilities of each entity are clear.

Where the experience is not faculty-led, the responsibilities of each entity vis-à-vis the project work are more complex. The host institution may propose the project based on an assessment of their needs, and the host institution's personnel may provide direct oversight of the project. However, the home institution is still responsible for general oversight of the students' work. It is the faculty leader of the home institution who must ensure that as the project progresses, the students continue to work within the scope of practice appropriate for their level of preparation. The home institution faculty will also need to monitor the progress of the project in relation to the length of the experience to ensure that the students are able to meet course requirements in a reasonable timeline and that the project meets any relevant home institution requirements for graduation. This monitoring requires regular contact with the students by email or telephone and periodic discussions with host institution personnel and, if necessary, a site visit to review the project. It is essential that home institution faculty members have established relationships and lines of communication with host site personnel so that any concerns regarding the quality of the experience can be quickly addressed and openly discussed. Equally, host site personnel need to feel comfortable in bringing issues to the home institution faculty if there are concerns about student participation or behavior.

Supervision of Students and the Use of Reflection

Beyond the oversight of the project as previously discussed, overall supervision of the students is a major part of home faculty responsibility. This includes monitoring students' health and safety, ensuring the flow of events and experiences for the students, and, importantly, helping the students develop awareness of their own responses to the experience and insights into the meaning of what they are experiencing. This last occurs through the use of reflection, which is an integral part of the service-learning experience. It is the process of reflection that moves the experience beyond the scope of a travel tour or a series of tasks, and reflection is where much of the real work of learning – that is, synthesis and integration of new learning into the existing paradigm – occurs.

Formal reflection exercises can take written or oral form, and can be carried out individually or in a group. When the experience is faculty-led, the process of reflection may occur in a group setting, with students exchanging reactions and insights. The faculty leader may use "prompts" to focus the group thinking in a specific direction, or may allow the students to bring forward the issues that are most relevant at the moment. Each strategy has value. Using prompts can help the students integrate their experiences with previous learning through coursework or reading. Prompts may also help students focus on issues that are uncomfortable or difficult for them to verbalize but are central to their full understanding of the experience. An "unacceptable" feeling that "I don't like these people" can be re-framed as they begin to recognize that "I am afraid," or "I am confused," or "I don't understand why...." It is also useful to have students reflect on their experience at times without prompts. While prompts direct the students' attention to specific issues, open reflection allows the student to explore areas the faculty leader may not have identified.

Reflection is most useful when it is used episodically throughout the experience.

Reflection at the end of the experience is essential but may not capture the feelings and responses that occur early on and throughout the experience. Structuring-in reflection exercises at the beginning of the experience, at the end, and at intervals throughout will help the student recognize his or her own process of personal change and growth over time. It is also important for faculty leaders to respond to the reflection, providing the student with reinforcement, or reframing and clarifying.

Debriefing and Evaluation

A final step in the implementation of a global service-learning program is to evaluate the experience from multiple perspectives. The process should include feedback from student participants and host institution participants, as well the home institution's faculty. Factors evaluated should include:

A. Did the experience meet the objectives of the course or curriculum?

B. What should have been different?

C. What worked and should continue?

D. What could be added or enhanced to improve the experience?

E. Did the site work and should it continue to be used?

F. Were the students optimally prepared for the experience? If not, what could be done better?

G. What recommendations would you make for the next experience?

In addition, if students have been in different settings for their experience, it is also useful to use the debriefing session to do some cross cultural comparison. Exercises may include contrasting different health care delivery systems, such as national health systems with the U.S. private-payer system. This time is also an opportunity for students to compare cultural understandings of what constitutes health and illness and perceptions of when health care should be sought. They may begin to explore some of the antecedents of health disparities by comparing, for example, beliefs about diabetes, health care seeking behaviors, and available resources in an urban environment in a southwestern state and an Indian reservation twenty miles away. While this exercise may not be structured formally as a reflection, it is a valuable learning activity.

Summary

Global service-learning is a valuable learning strategy for nurse educators. It provides opportunities for students to:

- increase their comfort and competence in the delivery of health care to diverse populations;

- deepen their understanding of the interrelationships between culture, community, and health;

- explore the antecedents of health disparities; and

- gain insights into the strengths and weaknesses of our health care delivery system.

The success of a global service-learning experience depends on extensive preliminary planning, careful negotiation with the host site, thoughtful selection and preparation of the students prior to leaving, and establishing protocols for ongoing monitoring and supervision throughout the experience. The use of reflection is essential to supervising the students' experience and enhancing their learning. Finally, the ongoing maintenance of a global service-learning partnership requires clear and regular communication and openness from both partners.

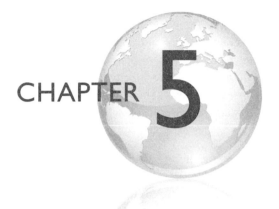

CHAPTER 5

Faculty-Administration Partnerships: Vital for Learning

Anne R. Bavier
E. Carol Polifroni
Kathryn Stewart Hegedus
Karen R. Breitkreuz

With advice from Jill Espelin, Lisa Marie Griffiths, Arthur Engler, John McNulty, Ross Lewin, and Kay Thurn.

As technology shrinks the world, our School joins our University's commitment to preparing students for global citizenship and global-marketplace careers, while supporting their growth into reflective, concerned, contributing members of the global community. Hallmarks of success in these efforts include growing flexibility and empathy in adapting to different communication styles, behaviors and cultural environments, based on growing respect for and ease in the diversity of cultures that are new to them, alongside growing curiosity, and strengthened ability to tolerate ambiguity and uncertainty. Underlying all of these is our students' growing ability to develop open, true, and lively human relationships with people from other cultures, including mutual learning and teaching. (University of Connecticut, Global Citizenship Curriculum Committee) http://globalcitizenship.uconn.edu/documents/global_learning_outcomes.pd.

In traditional academic models, the faculty has three essential areas of responsibility: the curriculum; students; and decisions about academic positions (the selection of new faculty, tenure, and promotion). Academic administrators are responsible for providing the infrastructure that faculty members need to succeed: finances, budgeting, hiring, legal contracts for clinical placement, licensure verification, and accreditation. The responsibilities of the two are interdependent, but different. A partnership with good communication is needed if the institution is to run smoothly. For example, an administrator cannot finalize clinical-placement contracts without the faculty's detailed plans for who will teach what. These partnerships are critical in study abroad (outside the U.S.) and study away (inside the U.S./territories) programming, which need seamless teamwork between faculty and administrative decision-makers.

The University of Connecticut School of Nursing (hereafter, the School) offers a model whereby faculty and administration work together to create meaningful, constructive study abroad/study away programs for nursing students. Through the years, our study abroad/away programming has grown, steadily and strategically. Ten years ago, we began with credible programs abroad that offered meaningful summer experiences and some academic credit to a few graduate and undergraduate students. Today, we offer undergraduates a full semester abroad/away, which features full classroom schedules, full clinical placements, and full-load course credits that parallel those that their classmates are earning on campus.

The chapter that follows was written jointly by two members of the UConn faculty (Hegedus and Breitkreuz) and two members of the administration (Bavier and Polifroni). We offer insights from our own experiences setting up and running a number of study abroad/away programs, particularly one in Cape Town, South Africa, which will be described in some detail.

Organizing Principles and Values

With a goal of 30 percent of undergraduate nursing students participating in study abroad/away, we began our efforts to establish study abroad/away programs by working to clarify our priorities, chiefly through analysis of other institutions' study abroad experiences and outcomes. Over time, we learned that study abroad/away has a long history of collaboration within academe and across borders; students often earn full academic credit while abroad/away; home faculty members sometimes but not always travel with and teach study abroad/away students; and not all placements are equal, since they are founded on various nations' and universities' standards and interpretations of academic excellence. We also learned that in many programs, cost is an insurmountable barrier to participation by some otherwise well-qualified students.

UConn's faculty and administration agreed that our programs would be predicated on the six guiding principles of our School's own long-established PRAXIS philosophy:

- **P**rofessionalism in behavior, presentation, and conduct;
- **R**espect for others, richness, and diversity, and self;
- **A**ccountability for actions;
- **X**cellence in research, practice, teaching and service;
- **I**ntegrity and inquisitiveness;
- **S**ervice to students, the profession and community.

In addition, we identified a number of program-specific study abroad organizing principles and goals. These include:

- nurturing long-term relationships with academic institutions/clinical-practice sites to assure respect and excellence in teaching and service, as essential for ongoing flexibility and growth;
- maintaining high university standards that respond to standards of our state's Board of Nursing Education (e.g., licensure, student-faculty ratios, faculty qualifications);
- assuring programming respectful of students' need to graduate on schedule and funding sources to open program participation to any otherwise-qualified student;
- selecting students on the basis of faculty assessments of their academic excellence and integrity;
- expecting ethical, professional student behavior at all times, consistent with the university's student conduct code;

- emphasizing global awareness and cultural knowledge in all program experiences, including students' responsibility to share what have learned both in-country and, later, at home; and

- refining and revising our program on the basis of formative and summative evaluations.

Faculty Roles and Responsibilities

Selection of Placements

For more than a decade, one of us (Hegedus), as a member of the School of Nursing faculty, has built an extensive network of international nursing connections while traveling and participating in international education forums, as input for our School's eventual expansion of study abroad opportunities. For example, she joined the North American Consortium of Nursing and Allied Health for International Cooperation (NACNAH), which works collaboratively with its European counterpart, the Consortium of Institutes of Higher Education in Health and Rehabilitation in Europe (COHEHRE). Her dedicated efforts saw their first dividends when we sent our first groups of carefully selected students to short-term summer programs abroad. For instance, for several summers, we sent undergraduates to an international health care course in Denmark (since closed). Academic credit was transferrable and, upon their return, the students were meticulously debriefed. This experience made it clear that faculty members could identify learning and cultural experiences abroad that would be consistent with our university's academic standards, and would be meaningful for participating nursing students. Now some seniors attend an eight-nation short course on end-of-life care in Belgium; their work is credited as alternate assignments in their capstone courses.

As our School's faculty members investigated programs with potential for our nursing students, our institution launched its own university-wide Office of Study Abroad, to systematically forge more and stronger university-to-university partnerships with institutions in other countries. Our faculty met with faculty from other schools and colleges within our university to exchange ideas and experiences, and to identify promising partner institutions. As faculty members joined our institution, additional well-functioning partnerships were established, including one in Cape Town, South Africa.

Our School has a particular dedication to serving vulnerable populations. Still, our faculty pondered whether the needs of Cape Town might be too intense for nursing undergraduates in a full-semester study abroad experience. Administrators invited a faculty "scout" (Hegedus) to visit Cape Town, to meet with a Study Abroad Office host coordinator (a Cape Town citizen), and to tour potential clinical-placement sites (e.g., an NGO that cares for orphans, or local nurse-managed health clinics serving impoverished neighborhoods). She visited housing where current university students lived and faculty quarters located nearby. By her assessment, Cape Town was a suitable site for our undergraduates' study abroad experiences. Clinical and theory objectives for maternal-child health and pediatrics could successfully be met there, and the site would offer exceptional opportunities to experience nursing in a different health care culture, with roles and responsibilities for nurses that were dramatically different from those at home.

It might have been luck that made us so fierce about assuring that every program feature and detail be checked and double-checked long before the students arrived in September. The faculty member appointed to lead their semester-long adventure arrived in Cape Town the preceding June. She reported to us regularly as planned. However, she had little faith in the program's partnerships, and she felt that the arrangements which had been made for logistics, transportation to and participation in various sites would take years to develop before they could be trusted. From her perspective, our program was not nearly ready to educate our nursing students. At her request, we brought her home early, debriefed her thoroughly, thanked her for her opinions, and assigned her to different courses.

Administrative and faculty leaders met to revisit our guiding principles and seriously to consider the implications if the former leader's assessments were accurate. We consulted in depth with the head of the university's Study Abroad Office, whose viewpoints were particularly pertinent since it was he who had opened the university's Cape Town program. He knew its host coordinator long and well. He judged the former leaders' opinions to be unduly gloomy or mistaken, and encouraged us to forge ahead. We did. A talented (and sunny) faculty member was appointed to lead the School's first study abroad semester in Cape Town. It was a brilliantly successful, life-changing adventure for our first cohort of students.

Each year since 2008, 12 to 16 of our senior nursing students have spent a full fall semester in Cape Town, where they fulfill School requirements in maternal-child care and pediatrics. In respectful regard for our state's Board of Nursing Education requirements, faculty members accompany them to Cape Town to provide required didactic and clinical content, sharing some classes with a local university. Faculty and students have formed mutually satisfying partnerships and friendships with the staff and clients at several clinical sites. Our students take courses in South African culture and history taught by local faculty members. Carefully selected field trips provide important visual and historical context (e.g., students visit the Robben Island prison where Nelson Mandela spent his many years of incarceration).

With program success proved by all stated and pertinent measures, faculty members began to suggest other locales to which our study abroad program might expand. A faculty member who had led a brief, pilot study away trip to San Juan, Puerto Rico, made a compelling case. Among the attractions of the San Juan site: Since most of our graduates practice in our state, our students would have cultural and linguistic advantages, because many Puerto Ricans now live and work in our area of the northeast. Administrators and faculty selected San Juan as our next focus area.

Our School has strong ties with the Veterans Administration System, which pointed us to investigating the local Veterans Administration Hospital in San Juan. Care is provided in both Spanish and English, and our nursing students and faculty were welcomed. Each fall semester, 10 to 12 students now study psychiatric-mental health and medical-surgical nursing in San Juan.

As faculty members have returned and shared their experiences, others have come to understand the administration's dedication to supporting, improving and expanding our School's study abroad offerings. They are tapping their own connections to create new, high-quality opportunities for our students. In a highly competitive faculty hiring market, the opportunity to work with our international program can be a deciding factor in employment decisions by prospective new hires. Moreover, the study abroad bug has spread to other, graduate-level tracks within the School. Our master's entry in nursing program (graduate entry into our profession for those who hold baccalaureate degrees in other academic disciplines) will take its first group to Haiti in the summer of 2012. Planning is under way for study abroad experiences for DNP candidates, too, with the first group going to England in the summer of 2012.

Selection of Students

We were fortunate that Cape Town was our first study abroad site. Cape Town's host coordinator visits our university each fall, to help interview and select students for the Cape Town program. He is deeply experienced in spotting students who are likely to succeed and thrive in a study abroad experience (and those who are not), and has been generous in sharing that acumen with us. In fact, our faculty now uses his approach in selecting students for all our study abroad/away experiences.

Clearly, only students in good academic standing are eligible even to apply. A written application is required – an adaptation (now including health care goals and issues) of the form used by our university's College of Liberal Arts and Sciences. While some questions are straightforward (e.g., "Have you ever traveled outside the U.S.?"), students are also asked to write essays explaining their professional goals. Following the written application, candidates are interviewed in a relaxed manner, typically by the Cape Town host coordinator (for the South Africa program) and two faculty members. The interviewers have key points to assess: Are the student's expectations realistic? Would the study abroad experience be relevant to the student's past activities and future goals? What is the student's tolerance for ambiguity and respect for cultural variations?

When all interviews are complete, the group ranks a preliminary list of students whom they recommend for the experience, alongside a list of those whose applications are denied. Then these lists are shared with coordinators of the pre-licensure courses, who often know the students well and may have relevant information (e.g., this student's mother is now terminally ill, or that student is solid academically but has an occasional history of disrespectful interactions with others). Rarely has the list been modified as a result of these discussions, but it is a final safety check before acceptances are published. Placements are offered to the top 12 to16 students for the Cape Town program and the top 10 to 12 for the San Juan experience; a waiting list includes approved students ranked below them. Typically, one or two successful applicants might withdraw, usually for personal/family reasons or failure to maintain the required grade-point average. Their places are offered to waiting-list students who still qualify.

Our faculty finds it difficult to reject any application for an outstanding opportunity like those described here. These are students they care for and know well. And our faculty is so passionately certain that a study abroad/away experience can deepen both the careers and the characters of participants, they would welcome the opportunity to approve every application! Denials generally are related to student attitude. For example, it is a deal-breaker if a student seeks the experience because "it'll look great on my resume." If a student expects the "study" part of study abroad to be a merely secondary objective or afterthought, that student will stay home. If the student exhibits behaviors (either within or outside nursing courses) that challenge standards of professionalism and respect, or reveals extreme fear and anxiety (as distinct from wholesome uncertainty) about personal safety or an ability to meet requirements, both the student and the group will be better served without that student in the program.

Orientation of Students and Families

Faculty members and administrators agree that students' families are an essential part of our School community; their contributions and confidence are among our keys to success. During the spring term, we invite families of students who will study abroad the following fall to join us for a reception. A short program includes a welcome from the administration, and distribution of contact details for senior faculty and administrators who will serve as families' resources and contacts while the students are away. We explain details of the provisions made for students' safety and health by the School and by the university's Study Abroad Office. Faculty members who will accompany the students are introduced, followed by brief remarks from faculty members who have led previous programs. We make it abundantly clear that administrators steadfastly support all faculty decisions regarding any student's professional behavior and compliance with the Student Code of Conduct. On-site faculty members are authorized to dismiss any student at any time, for cause. It is important for all concerned to understand that the administration and faculty speak with one voice in these actions and decisions. Students who are sent home are to be referred to the Student Conduct Board, which has authority to expel such students from the university. To date, no such action has been necessary. But families actually find our no-nonsense stance is comforting. Communication channels are open, and families and faculty alike enjoy meeting each other.

Program Evaluation

For the first two years of the Cape Town program, we engaged in extensive debriefing of each student and faculty member, and we made a number of program refinements on the basis of those debriefings. For example, students wanted to celebrate Thanksgiving by inviting people to whom they were grateful – local nurses and others who had helped them – to share their American holiday feast. This was an easy program addition, and a meaningful one for our students. Students wanted their semester's academic work to be completed and submitted before they returned to the U.S., so the due-date for a paper in pediatric nursing was moved to antedate their return home. Issues about housing and classroom spaces were identified and resolved.

At first, the student and faculty debriefings took the form of written and oral narratives. Faculty members determined that a more structured evaluation was needed to determine if goals were met relating to global citizenship and cultural awareness. One faculty member (Breitkreuz) developed a systematic evaluation to address key questions. For instance: What were the students' initial (pre-program) readiness levels for cross-cultural adaptation, and how do they compare with final (post-program) levels of socio-cultural adaptation and satisfaction? Were our cultural learning activities useful in advancing students' and faculty members' attitudes and abilities in cross-cultural development? What was the final, overall satisfaction of the students and faculty members with their study abroad experiences? A socio-cultural adaptation scale and other established instruments are now used to conduct this ongoing study, within parameters designed to protect human subjects (e.g., informed consent and not evaluating a group until all course grades for the term are finalized).

Some faculty members reported that at times they felt lonely and isolated from colleagues while they were away. Another "easy fix" for our joint faculty-administration partnership, in this technological age. We simply equipped faculty computers with webcams and Skype accounts to simplify overseas faculty members' communication with colleagues. In addition, regular conferences were scheduled with a member of the administration to convey School news (like the final approval of a new building addition), to help faculty make/execute plans for their future assignments (like ordering books for the upcoming term), and simply to chat together "over coffee." Study abroad faculty veterans continued their peer support, begun in pre-departure orientation, via regular dialogue with those on-site. These conversations allowed an overseas faculty member to keep us abreast of study abroad program news (large and small), while they learned more about what was happening with the students who remained at home.

Faculty members also reported that it was difficult for them to provide all required course content (8.5 credits), even for their small groups. Their problem was not our nursing curriculum, which requires concurrent clinical practice and related didactic coursework; those elements were typically well within their expertise and experience. Their challenge was (and is) the required extra-nursing course material (e.g., leadership), which, on campus, is typically taught by different faculty members. For courses taught in a time zone close to ours in the U.S., teachers are accustomed to using an interactive television to broadcast among our five campuses. That is a realistic option for a site like Puerto Rico. Such simultaneous instruction is impossible, however, between our main campus and Cape Town, which is six hours ahead of Connecticut. So faculty members have adopted a different pedagogical approach, moving into a seminar format with assigned readings, instead of a lecture-discussion approach.

Before their departure, the faculty members gather each student group for simulation exercises to give the students practice with skills to be introduced in the upcoming course. This is challenging for the students, because they have not yet studied the relevant didactic content. Using university-approved professional-development funds (supplemented by her own checkbook), the director of our Clinical Simulation Laboratories traveled to Cape Town to conduct a postpartum hemorrhage simulation at the local hospital. The director served as "patient," and overseas faculty members were responsible for set-up and debriefing. Then, the two faculty members together repeated the simulation for local hospital staff, demonstrating our commitment to sharing our experience and knowledge with our hosts, and advancing our commitment to the guiding principle of forming long-term relationships.

Administration Roles and Responsibilities

The main contributions of academic administrators in setting up a study abroad/away program are related to providing all necessary resources for faculty and students. Of course, administrators are in charge of the finances. But there is a great deal more to operating a successful study abroad program than simply coming up with the money. One key is administrators' responsibility to provide for fulfillment of the guiding principles outlined above.

Administrative Agreements

Typically, a nursing school executes a memorandum of understanding with each agency where students fulfill their clinical-practice requirements. The agreement identifies the responsibilities of each institution regarding student placements. These evolving documents are founded on long-term relationships between institutional administrators and educators. Refinements are instituted cordially, with a presumption of good will, and with general understanding of the challenges each faces. As a public university, we work closely with our state attorney general's office to review and refine agreement modifications. An agreement with a clinical agency in a foreign nation brings a new set of challenges, however. For example, our state's laws require that agreements contain specific language about diversity, open competition, etc. Even organizations in neighboring states sometimes find these terms challenging. Our state recognizes no exceptions to these terms, even with international parties.

Consequently, clinical agencies in another nation must have their own legal counsel meticulously review the agreement's language for conflicts with that nation's own laws. It is virtually impossible to predict the timeline required to accomplish these tasks. At our university, administrators prefer to send faculty members, the people who will actually be on-site as the work evolves, to hammer out details through discussions with their future partners. It is our belief that these front-line relationships are the foundation of new partnerships that will become long-term relationships. However, international partners may prefer to forge such agreements only with high-level administrative representatives, rather than with faculty members. The budgeting implications are clear.

At UConn, new-site development budgets now include costs for faculty-faculty dialogue, with our faculty charged with assessing potential. If needed, expenses will be budgeted for an administrator to travel to the new site to finalize arrangements. Because our faculty is experienced and knowledgeable about our courses and guiding principles, this looks to us like an unnecessary expenditure of time and money. But if it saves a promising learning adventure for future students, it is worthwhile.

In some instances, agreements with a partner academic institution allow student placements in their affiliated clinical agencies. Regardless, attention to affiliate clinical sites is important.

Special Nursing Issues Related to Travel Abroad

Our university's Office of Study Abroad is a significant resource. Its team guides students and faculty through matters such as international health insurance, and offers a group policy that is both comprehensive and cost-effective. However, host country regulations related to foreign students vary considerably from country to country. For example, the

Nursing Council in South Africa requires an opportunity to approve specific lists of students and faculty members who will be in the country, and approval requires that UConn acquire specific student/faculty insurance for the listed individuals. Notice must be given no later than five months in advance, and the invoice must be paid and receipt documented prior to students and faculty entering the country. The collaboration has been facilitated by our faculty visiting with nursing leaders in Cape Town. However, the regulations mandate that our selection of students and faculty be final the April before their September arrival.

Housing

Faculty and students need to be housed separately. Finding and renting appropriate housing is relatively simple in an established university program, like ours in South Africa, where the host coordinator selects the housing and the Study Abroad Office leases and furnishes it. In addition, a host resident advisor hired through that office manages all relevant facets of student life, including the typical "dorm" meetings, food purchasing assignments, and the like.

But locales that lack a seasoned host coordinator may require a great deal more administrative attention. At one point during our first year in Puerto Rico, our dean determined that the students' housing was no longer appropriate since the landlord continued to fail to make agreed-upon changes. She (Bavier) re-located the students to a hotel. The School absorbed the additional costs, an unexpected but necessary budget item.

Students also need housing support when they return to campus. During their semesters away, their dorm rooms have been reassigned. The university provides a dormitory, Global House, which houses visiting and returning students. The administration alerts the Department of Residential Life concerning how many students will be returning and requiring such housing.

Costs

Student fees for the semester are calculated to cover travel; lodging (though not food); insurance; university tuition; a Study Abroad Office administrative service fee (currently $475 per student); and local cultural experiences (to assist students in developing an appropriate understanding of the host environment) and faculty costs. All funds are paid to the Study Abroad Office, which disperses program funds. In order to meet local expenses (e.g., cultural excursions, rental cars for faculty members, drivers for student outings), the faculty members on-site sets up a bank account for funds advanced through the Study Abroad Office. Faculty members document all expenditures, and unspent funds are returned at the end of the program.

For reasons of both good will and expediency, faculty and administrators try to be flexible, too. When our students' Puerto Rican landlord was having trouble with the electricity and water bills, we agreed that our on-site faculty member would pay the utility bills and charge back those costs. When it became truly burdensome to keep up with multiple local charges, that experiment was not repeated. Faculty members are authorized to act on unexpected expenses, too – with discernment. For example, one cultural excursion included a local religious institution. While there was no admission charge, clearly there was expectation of a "donation." The faculty member had full license to make that on-site donation, although it was unanticipated and unbudgeted.

Financial Aid and Scholarships

An unfortunate aspect of the study abroad billing system is that it shows no separate line-item figure for tuition. This has complicated some families' efforts to validate loans made on the basis of tuition bills. Our administrators routinely write individual letters to affected families to document that the student's course work is equivalent to that taught in the U.S. and is taught by qualified university faculty. Some loan programs refuse support for study abroad, so students and their families must find other sources. Some scholarships have similar limitations regarding funding study abroad; in such cases the dean works diligently to secure necessary funds from private philanthropy. To date, funds have been secured for some students in our South Africa program.

As they prepare to apply for study abroad/away programs, aspirants are encouraged to attend information sessions with our International Coordinator (Hegedus), who presents program requirements and details, including pertinent financial considerations. Students then are expected to raise and resolve these issues with their families, long before the selection process is underway.

Faculty selection

As described above, the faculty member assigned to lead our first Cape Town semester was not a good fit. Had this not become clear in time for us to replace her, our Cape Town programming might well have failed completely, failing our pioneering students at the same time. Clearly, the administrators involved had a lot to learn about the qualities needed to make a study abroad experience successful; the right faculty leader brings more than good teaching evaluations and a desire to go abroad. We talked with a humanities professor who regularly takes students to Cape Town about her expectations and experiences. She taught us more than operational details. She made clear that the faculty leader needs to be a flexible person, willing to see unanticipated events as opportunities to learn about the culture and to develop awareness and respect in students.

With that insight, our administrators now seek faculty with track records in similar types of endeavors, such as faculty members who have opened new clinical placement sites or launched interdisciplinary collaborations. For both Cape Town and San Juan, we have an established rotation of faculty. While our faculty members report they have loved their study abroad adventures, they prefer not to go every academic year. (They are delighted to go every two or three years, however.)

Staffing for study abroad/away programming requires that the School hire adjuncts as replacements for those traveling. However, returning faculty weave the experience into subsequent courses so that more students receive the benefit of their experiences with other cultures. Administrators and faculty alike believe this is a worthy investment.

Faculty Compensation

Our Office of Study Abroad calculates student charges to include funds for the School to support adjunct faculty as replacements. These funds are appreciated, but are calculated at the university's standard rate for adjuncts across disciplines. Nursing adjuncts, who teach clinical courses, are in such high demand that they are compensated at a rate significantly higher than those in other disciplines because of fierce local market competition. The dean must anticipate and budget for these additional costs.

The study abroad/away faculty role does not include management of the student residence or typical issues that arise in a dormitory setting. As the senior person present, however, the on-site faculty member does become involved when issues fall outside the scope of the host resident advisor. The faculty leader also works with the host coordinator to fine-tune schedules for cultural experiences (e.g., avoiding the weekends just before major papers are due). Within the faculty's union contract, no mechanism exists to provide supplemental pay for such services. In recognition of the extra demands on the time of faculty leaders, the dean provides them with professional-development funding.

Conclusion

UConn has created and implemented a study abroad/away program that meets our guiding principles and upholds the School's PRAXIS philosophy. Importantly, we would not have succeeded without the strong support and focused teamwork of both faculty members and administrators, each understanding, supporting, and respecting the work of the other. We look down the road together. All team members offer suggestions and thoughts to make our program better.

A consistent feature of all our current sites is the ability to provide clinical-practice courses. We recognize that this may not be true in all future endeavors. Faculty members are beginning to discuss program designs for shorter experiences that might be folded into existing courses, including the welcoming of pre-licensure students from other nations. In addition, historically, faculty exchanges have been arranged by individuals with colleagues in other nations. Now, we are developing systematic exchanges with two universities to provide a forum for joint scholarly development.

Administrators and faculty members together have made great strides in developing our study abroad/away opportunities, all with an eye toward preparing a cadre of nurses capable of contributing more than their share to the health care needs of the global community. It is essential work. It is an important partnership.

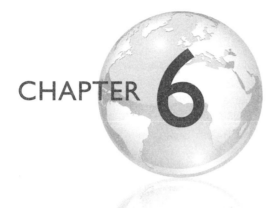

CHAPTER 6

Host Institution Perspectives

Lynda Law Wilson
Doreen Harper

Globalization challenges nurses, as the largest group of health care providers, to be mindful of the many factors that influence health care across the world, including social, environmental, economic, and cultural determinants of health, new and emerging diseases, and resources to address health needs (Memmott et al., 2010). International exchange and educational programs can increase nurses' cultural competence, enhance education and service, and address global health issues (Lange & Ailinger, 2001; Leinonen, 2006). Such programs also offer opportunities to promote scholarship for both the host institution and international participants.

In this chapter, we will discuss factors that should be considered by a host institution that receives international nurses as part of an exchange or educational program using a service-learning partnership approach, with the University of Alabama at Birmingham School of Nursing (UABSON) serving as an example. The UABSON is a Pan American Health Organization (PAHO)/World Health Organization (WHO) Collaborating Center for International Nursing, or WHOCC – that is, an institution designated by the Director-General of WHO to form part of an inter-institutional collaborative network established to further the goals and mission of the WHO, and to help address global health needs by sharing information, services, research, and educational programs (WHO, 2011). There are currently 42 Nursing and Midwifery WHOCCs, and many of these centers participate in international exchange or educational programs.

The International Nursing Leadership Program (INLP) at the UABSON – the formal name for our international nursing exchange program – lasts about three weeks and focuses on global public health leadership development, with an opportunity for participants to strengthen their English-language skills. The program was initiated in 2006 and is offered every other year. The first two programs were open to nurses from any Latin American country. The first set of participants, in 2006, comprised 13 nurses from Chile; the second, in 2008, included 18 nurses from Brazil, Chile, Colombia, and Honduras. The 2010 INLP was expanded to also include nurses from Zambia, where the UABSON had initiated several ongoing partnerships and collaborative projects. That year saw the largest program yet, with 25 participating nurses coming from Brazil, Chile, Costa Rica, Honduras, Peru, and Zambia.

The framework used in this chapter to organize the discussion of host institution responsibilities is the Regis Model for Strategic Planning (Carty & White, 1996; Chinoy, 1993). The Regis Model was developed by The Regis Group (TRG), a management consulting practice based in Virginia.

Partner Roles and Responsibilities: Overview of the Regis Model

International exchange and educational programs offered by nursing schools are based on reciprocal partnerships among educational institutions, health care organizations, nongovernmental organizations (NGOs), and communities. The Regis Model for Strategic Planning offers a means by which the host institution and its international partners can work together in the assessment, planning, implementation, and evaluation of such a program. Carty and White (1996) described the application of the Regis Model in developing an international exchange program, noting that the model has been extensively used by educational institutions and by Nursing and Midwifery WHOCCs in the PAHO region.

For the purpose of this chapter, the Regis model has been adapted to include the following components: (a) identification of the program mission and vision; (b) assessment of the group and current environment; (c) identification of goals and objectives; (d) development of strategies and a tactical plan; and (e) evaluation and planning for a cyclical review process. These components, as applied to international exchange and educational programs, are described in the following sections.

Identification of the Program Mission and Vision

The first step in any service-learning program or global collaboration is to identify the program's mission and vision, and to ensure that they match the mission and goals of the host institution and its collaborating partners (Immonen, Anderssen, & Lvova, 2008; Memmott et al., 2010). Involvement of all key players in preliminary discussions of the proposal is critical to ensure a sustainable and successful program. When these exchanges are offered by institutions with a Nursing and Midwifery WHOCC, the initial planning often begins by discussing the program with the WHO regional nursing advisor and including the program as an activity listed in the terms of reference and objectives for the Center.

The INLP is included as a key activity in the terms of reference for the WHOCC at the UABSON, and is consistent with the mission and goals of the school. For example, the UABSON has formulated its mission as follows: "The UABSON, as part of a research university and academic health center, prepares nurse leaders to excel as clinicians, researchers and educators; and advances knowledge and the delivery of high quality health care in Alabama and worldwide" (UABSON, 2011). It expresses its vision in this way: "To be a dynamic and innovative leader, raising the quality of health care and expanding the educated nursing workforce in Alabama and worldwide" (UABSON, 2011).

Assessment of the Group and Current Environment

If the project is an educational program, potential participants may not be identified until after the program is developed and advertised. However, it is important at the outset to conduct a needs assessment to identify interest in the program among potential participants or collaborators (Immonen et al., 2008; Memmott et al., 2010). The preliminary needs assessment should also address any strengths, weaknesses, opportunities and threats that might impact the project. Assessment of the group and current environment also requires an analysis of the administrative structure within the host institution for organizing and coordinating the program. If the host institution is a school of nursing within a larger university, assessment of support services within the school and the university would also be helpful (e.g., Study Away Office, International Student and Scholar Office, School of Nursing Office of Student Affairs, Office of International Programs, etc.).

Immonen et al. (2008) identified five potential challenges in planning cross-national project work and collaboration that might be considered in assessing the group and current environment: (a) cultural differences; (b) language differences; (c) the role of the participating organizations in their respective societies; (d) technology; and (e) logistical concerns. Each of these areas was considered in the planning and design of the INLP. For example, in planning the 2010 INLP, the organizers considered cultural and language differences between participants from Zambia and Latin American countries, and the program was expanded so the Zambian nurses could attend seminars offered by the Sparkman Center for Global Health while the Latin American nurses participated in English classes. The program coordinator also worked closely with partners in Zambia and in Latin America, as well as with UAB faculty, in planning the program and incorporating opportunities for discussion of specific leadership challenges so that participants had opportunities to learn from one another.

Identification of Program Goals and Objectives

Data from the initial assessment is used to refine and shape the program's goals and objectives. Open communication among participants and with potential collaborators in the host institution is necessary to develop program goals and implementation plans. In the Regis Model, goals are defined as priority areas for ongoing program consideration and development, and objectives are measurable targets to be accomplished. When identifying program goals and objectives, it is important to consider the resources that are available and that will be required, including human and financial resources, time, space, equipment, and community partners. Byrne (1998) noted that when considering human resources it is important to ensure that the host institution has the expertise to address the program participants' needs. Other factors to consider include overhead costs, which must be taken into account in planning the program budget; liability and health insurance for program participants; security issues; assistance with travel arrangements and housing for participants; and local cultural attractions that should be incorporated into program plans.

Memmott et al. (2010) noted that international programs in schools of nursing cannot be sustainable without commitment of a group of faculty. In addition, ensuring sustainable program resources requires a commitment from the organization's administrative leadership. It takes a village to host an international education exchange program or service-learning project! One strategy that has been used to promote involvement of faculty at the UABSON in global initiatives is a specific goal in the school's strategic plan specifying that at least 30 percent of faculty members will contribute to the global mission of the school.

When collaborating partners have been identified in advance, it is also helpful to involve them in the initial assessment and planning process. Ross described a "hermanamiento" (sister school) method of collaboration between the schools of nursing at Duquesne University in Pennsylvania and the Polytechnic University in Managua, Nicaragua (Ross, 2000). In each school, a committee of faculty and students worked to plan and coordinate the program, and also sought funding to ensure its sustainability. Another strategy is appointing a council or group within the school or host institution to oversee all aspects of international program planning (Memmott et al., 2010).

The goals of the INLP have evolved over the three program offerings based on lessons learned, changing partner needs, and program evaluation data. The goals of the 2010 program were to (a) strengthen nursing leadership capacity; (b) enhance child and family health through innovative nursing care delivery programs; (c) enhance written and spoken English skills to promote leadership development; and (d) promote ongoing collaboration on projects to strengthen global nursing and health care delivery. The 2010 program had four different components, which were tailored to participants' individual learning needs:

1. Participants who were interested in improving their professional written and spoken English skills had the opportunity to attend classes at the UAB English Language and Culture Institute.

2. Participants who did not attend the English Institute classes attended seminars on global public health leadership offered at the UAB Sparkman Center for Global Health Summer Institute.

3. Each participant was assigned a faculty mentor/collaborator who worked with the participant to develop a plan for an individual leadership development project to be implemented during the year following the end of the three-week program in Alabama. Time was provided for participants to meet with the mentors and to arrange individualized activities such as library work or visits to health care facilities.

4. Finally, all participants took a course entitled "Global Perspectives in Nursing Leadership." UAB undergraduate and graduate students were also invited to register for the course as an elective.

Development of Strategies and a Tactical Plan

The fourth stage in the model involves developing specific strategies and plans to be implemented before, during, and after the program.

Prior to the program. Issues related to logistics and to the recruitment and selection of program participants are among those that must be considered prior to offering the program.

Recruitment and selection of program participants. Criteria for recruiting and selecting participants should be identified based on the program's mission, goals, and objectives. It is important to consider factors such as language skills and the professional, educational, and experiential background of prospective participants in order to ensure that there is a match between participants' needs and expectations and the program offered. It is critical to allow sufficient time between the notification of selected applicants and the beginning of the program. At least three or four months will be needed for obtaining visas, making travel arrangements, securing health clearance, and arranging for leave from work and family responsibilities.

Logistical planning. Many factors must be considered by the host institution in planning the logistics to ensure a successful program. These include travel arrangements, housing, health issues, and budgets. Another key issue is the timing of the program, given differing academic and holiday schedules across global institutions.

Travel arrangements may be the responsibility of the host institution or the participants. In the latter case, arrangements are needed for meeting participants when they arrive in the host city, and emergency contact numbers should be provided in case of changes in airline schedules. If the host institution assumes responsibility for paying for participant travel, it is critical to include a contingency fund in the budget in the event of increases in airfares or other travel expenses. There are many types of housing arrangements including placing participants with host families, arranging housing on campus, or in local hotels. Housing with host families has advantages in terms of providing rich opportunities for cross-cultural learning, but it is critical to ensure that there is adequate orientation for both the participant and host family to ensure success of such arrangements.

There are many health issues that must be considered by the host institution. The host institution's regulations may require participants to submit a health history and document any special health needs that may arise during the program. The institution may also have requirements related to immunizations or screening for tuberculosis. In order to obtain visas to enter the United States for educational or cultural exchanges, visitors must document that they have adequate health insurance (defined by the U.S. Department of State). The host institution should identify local health providers who can address health needs of participants that may arise during the program.

Careful attention to budgetary issues is critical for the success of any international or service-learning program. The host institution should identify all program costs and ensure that funding is available either from the institution, external sources, or fees charged to participants. Such costs include costs of staff and faculty time; institutional overhead; meals and housing for participants; participant travel (both international and local); visa and SEVP (Student and Exchange Visitor Program) fees; health insurance; liability insurance; fees to cover programs, including visits to local cultural attractions; and other institutional fees. For example, if the program is housed at a university, there may be fees for participants to use the internet or computer resources, the library, or recreational facilities. One expense that is often overlooked is the overhead to the host institution, including expenses for both the host institution and program participants associated with communication (by fax, email, or phone calls) during planning for the program (Immonen et al., 2008).

Once program plans have been finalized, it is important to plan strategies for pre-departure orientation of program participants. These strategies may include preparation of a participant handbook; a narrated PowerPoint presentation or videotape that can be sent to participants or posted on a website; telephone conferences; or internet-based conferences using platforms such as Skype, Elluminate, or the Wimba Live Classroom. Such pre-departure orientation material should address the culture of the host country, provide information about program logistics and requirements, and include information about local contacts that can be shared with participants' family members so that they can be contacted easily in case of emergency.

During the program. When planning the program schedule, it is important to allow time for participants to recover from jet lag and fatigue following their travel. The program schedule, in general, should include unscheduled time where participants can network with each other and with their hosts. Over-scheduling can lead to burnout of both participants and hosts.

It is often helpful to use the first day of the program to provide an overall orientation, where participants can meet each other and their hosts and tour the host institution. Time on the first day can also be set aside to address outstanding logistical issues, such as obtaining university identification cards, documenting visa status with the institution's international office, reviewing health history forms, or providing proof of health and liability insurance coverage. Scheduling creative and fun "ice breaker" activities helps participants and hosts get to know one another and sets the stage for successful collaborations and partnerships.

A key issue to be considered when planning any program for international participants relates to language differences (Immonen et al., 2008). If the program will be conducted in English and English is not the participants' primary language, it will be important to include a basic level of English proficiency as a requirement for participation, or arrange for interpreters throughout all aspects of the program. Even if English language proficiency is included as a program prerequisite, it is often difficult to validate participants' level of proficiency prior to the beginning of the program. Some applicants may rate their level of proficiency as adequate, but find that they have problems comprehending the language once they arrive at the host institution. In some cases, participation in English language classes might be integrated as a component of the program. It may be helpful to have a faculty member who is fluent in the participants' language, and who can help the students adapt to the living and academic arrangements of the host institution (Ryan, Markowski, Ura, & Liu-Chiang, 1998). At the UABSON, the coordinator and the director of the INLP were fluent in English and Spanish, facilitating communication with the Latin American participants.

Sensitivity to and respect for cultural differences are critical for program success. There may be differences in communication patterns, time orientation, the meaning of gestures, food preferences, and dress among program participants and hosts (Immonen et al., 2008). In the INLP, international participants were encouraged to wear their traditional dress, and activities were arranged so that participants could share their foods and other cultural traditions with UABSON students and faculty. Immonen et al. (2008) described a cultural difference in communication and interaction patterns among participants in a cross-national collaboration in the arctic Barents region in Northern Europe (p. 845):

> In Russia, for example, it is thought impolite not to engage in some small talk before coming to the agreed agenda, whereas for Scandinavians, it is more customary to "not waste time." Thus, Russians may give an impression of avoiding the real issues while Scandinavians may give an impression of insensitivity and rudeness. In addition, Scandinavians have a more relaxed dress code, which may give the false impression that one does not appreciate one's partners.

It is often helpful to include discussion of cultural differences as part of the program, and to build in opportunities for participants to share their cultures and experiences. Having the participants live with host families and providing opportunities to visit local cultural attractions offers participants ways to learn about the culture of the host country. Hosts should also be sensitive to the challenges that visitors may face, including language barriers, separation from family and familiar foods and customs, cultural differences, and fears related to the need to succeed (Ryan et al., 1998). During the 2010 INLP, one of the Zambian participants indicated that he felt uncomfortable saying grace before meals with his host family, even though this was an important part of his mealtime at home. The coordinator plans to address this in future programs by encouraging both program participants and host families to honor one another's religious and cultural preferences and practices. Another example highlights the importance of sensitivity to cultural differences. When several of the Zambian participants in the 2010 INLP reported that they missed having "nchima," a corn meal product that is a stable component of the diet for many Zambians, their host family members found an African grocery store, purchased the corn meal, and then invited the Zambian guests to teach them how to prepare the food.

Allowing sufficient time for discussion, feedback, and de-briefing throughout the program will ensure that activities can be modified to address problems that may arise. It is also critical to ensure that participants have clear information about who to contact for any special needs or emergencies, including cell phone numbers of program coordinators in the event that issues arise after regular office hours, such as health emergencies or accidents.

After the program. An important component of many service-learning or international exchange programs is the opportunity to develop and maintain sustainable partnerships and collaborations. There are many models for such partnerships. For example, during the INLP, program participants partner with a faculty member to develop a special project or leadership development plan to be implemented once they return home. The increased availability of internet technology can facilitate such collaboration, although it must be recognized that there are potential limitations with technology. Internet may not be readily available in many countries, and even if it is available, the bandwidth may be relatively low, precluding the ability to access large files or use audio or video chat technology. Despite these challenges, technology has been used successfully by participants and faculty in the UAB program, and by others (Plummer & Nyang'au, 2009). Immonen et al. (2008) also noted a challenge with sharing resources on CDs or DVDs, which are often programmed to work in only one geographic region. Using these resources might require zone-free CD/DVD players, which are not always available.

Perhaps the greatest challenge to maintaining ongoing partnerships and collaborations after the end of the program relates to time constraints associated with distance, time zones, and other commitments on the part of the hosts as well as program participants, once the face-to-face components of the program are completed. Anticipating these constraints, and developing specific goals and expectations during the program, may help to minimize this barrier.

Evaluation and Planning for a Cyclical Review Process

The final component to be considered by a host institution involves planning for program evaluation and for a cyclical review process so that evaluation data can be used to improve future program offerings. If the evaluation data will be published or disseminated in a formal way, many institutions require approval by a research ethics committee or Institutional Review Board. It is helpful to collect evaluation data from multiple sources (e.g. hosts, participants, and participants' supervisors or colleagues), and to use a variety of data collection methods (e.g. surveys, interviews, and focus-group discussions). The INLP was evaluated by asking both program participants and faculty collaborators to complete surveys evaluating the leadership classes and overall program activities at the end of the program. In addition, email surveys were sent to both faculty and participants every two years after the end of the program to monitor progress on collaborative projects and communications. In some cases it may be appropriate (with prior consent of program participants) to survey participants' supervisors to evaluate the extent to which participation influenced their subsequent professional activities.

Collaborative Activities

Collaborative activities are based on the core components of service-learning and include developing meaningful and reciprocal relationships and engaging partners in preparation, planning, and resource management, as well as evaluation of the program. For example, initial collaboration for the UABSON International Nursing Leadership Program required extensive information-sharing, needs assessment, and ongoing communication to incorporate our global partners in setting and implementing the program agenda. We worked closely with PAHO/WHOCC representatives and with nursing colleagues around the world, including colleagues from other nursing and midwifery WHOCCs, universities, nursing schools, and health entities interested in international educational exchange programs. Among other things, we worked collaboratively to pursue financial support for the program.

Many different organizations can facilitate the establishment of collaborative inter-national exchange or educational programs. Besides the WHOCCs, these include faith-based groups and volunteer or nongovernmental organizations such as Rotary International (www.rotary.org/en/Pages/ridefault.aspx), Lions Clubs International (http://www.lionsclubs. org/EN/index.php), the Council for International Educational Exchanges (www.ciee.org), the Council for the International Exchange of Scholars (www.cies.org), or Partners of the Americas (www.partners.net). Collaborative partnerships bring together the numerous resources needed to support these international educational program exchanges. For example, the UABSON has collaborated with several NGOs to enable nurses from Central America to attend the International Nursing Leadership Program. Partners have helped with planning and developing the program as well as with recruiting and selecting program participants. This type of collaboration requires ongoing communication as the partners plan the program and arrange logistics.

Another aspect of collaboration is that between participants and students/faculty at the host institution before, during, and after the program. During the INLP, several special events were hosted to encourage student, faculty and community collaboration, such as a dinner recognizing the host families and their international guests. In addition, UABSON students were able to participate in the leadership program as a nursing elective course, allowing them to learn about global nursing and health care while remaining in Alabama.

Conclusion

In planning international exchange, educational, or service-learning programs, host institutions must collaborate with multiple partners and ensure that the program is based on an assessment of participants' needs, with mutual respect and recognition of the benefit for all parties. Using a framework such as the Regis Model can facilitate a systematic approach to program planning, implementation, and follow-up, and ensure that programs are successful and sustainable.

References

Byrne, M. W. (1998). Productive international faculty exchange: One Columbia University to Gothenburg University example. *Journal of Advanced Nursing, 27*(6), 1296–1304.

Carty, R. M., & White, J. F. (1996). Strategic planning for international education: The Regis Model. *Nursing Outlook, 44*(2), 89–93.

Chinoy, M. P. (1993). *The Regis Model: Strategic planning process.* Leesburg, Virginia: The Regis Group.

Immonen, I., Anderssen, N., & Lvova, M. (2008). Project work across borders in the arctic Barents region: Practical challenges for project members. *Nurse Education Today, 28*(7), 841–848.

Lange, I., & Ailinger, R. L. (2001). International nursing faculty exchange model: A Chile-USA case. *International Nursing Review, 48*(2), 109–116.

Leinonen, S. J. (2006). International nursing exchange programs. *Journal of Continuing Education in Nursing, 37*(1), 16-20.

Memmott, R. J., Coverston, C. R., Heise, B. A., Williams, M., Maughan, E. D., Kohl, J., & Palmer, S. (2010). Practical considerations in establishing sustainable international nursing experiences. *Nursing Education Perspectives, 31*(5), 298–302.

Plummer, C. A., & Nyang'au, T. O. (2009). Reciprocal e-mentoring: Accessible international exchanges. *International Social Work, 52*(6), 811–822. doi: 10.1177/0020872809342652

Ross, C. A. (2000). Building bridges to promote globalization in nursing: The development of a hermanamiento. *Journal of Transcultural Nursing, 11*(1), 64-67.

Ryan, D., Markowski, K., Ura, D., & Liu-Chiang, C.Y. (1998). International nursing education: Challenges and strategies for success. *Journal of Professional Nursing, 14*(2), 69–77. doi: Doi: 10.1016/s8755-7223(98)80033-1

University of Alabama at Birmingham School of Nursing. (2011). Mission, vision, core values, and strategic goals. Retrieved from http://www.uab.edu/nursing/about/mission-and-strategic-goals

World Health Organization. (2011). Collaborating centers. Retrieved from http://www.who.int/collaboratingcentres/cc_historical/en/index3.html

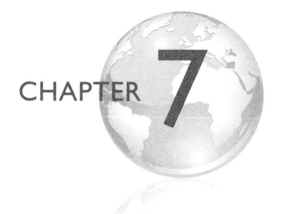

CHAPTER 7

Home and Host: Building a Partnership

Erin D. Maughan
Barbara A. Heise
Sheri Palmer
Mary Williams
Catherine R. Coverston

Underlying all global service-learning is a reciprocal relationship between the host community and the school of nursing (Bailey, Carpenter, & Harrington, 1999). Reciprocity allows for a win-win situation: the student benefits through experiential and reflective learning; and the host community benefits through knowledge and empowerment to meet their needs or, in the case of highly advanced health care systems, the opportunity to share health care accomplishments. Planning must ensure that both the needs of the community and the objectives of the academic course are met.

This chapter offers guidance in choosing a site and setting up a global service-learning (GSL) project, based on our experiences at the Brigham Young University College of Nursing. At the time of writing, the college runs about 10 different GSL programs, in places as far-flung as Ecuador, Finland, Ghana, India, Taiwan, and Tonga, as well as closer to home, in underserved rural communities and Native American communities in the United States. A case study drawn from our experience in Ecuador will close the chapter.

Choosing a Host Community

Selecting a Site

For an educational institution, the most crucial concern is to identify a site that will provide student experiences meeting the institution's stated goals and learning outcomes. A clear statement of objectives is key to program development and can help you stay focused as you explore and evaluate various opportunities. Whether your focus is developing cultural awareness, helping the students gain new skills and knowledge, or implementing projects suggested by the host community, clear objectives will help narrow your search. In this regard, since collaboration requires that both parties stand to gain, there needs to be a "give back" to the host community, which can occur through service-learning by the students. This service-learning experience can be as simple as helping to care for patients and helping out at health fairs to joint ventures in implementing evidence-based practice, research, or quality improvement projects identified by the host community.

Sustainability and capacity building are top priorities in selecting a host community because of the amount of time required to develop the site, including identifying key contacts. Returning to a site for at least three to five years can significantly decrease the burden of set-up over time and increase the likelihood of higher-level interactions each time you return, as you gain more knowledge of the host community and build stronger relationships. Sustainability and capacity building with a host community also allows us to build a relationship of trust where we can work together on a common goal. This is much preferred to having students visit strictly for an observation experience.

An option that makes set-up easier is partnering with other schools or colleges on campus, in areas such as public health, business, or engineering. Joint programs of this nature allow you to share the burdens of planning and logistics, and also help students learn to work in interdisciplinary teams, which can broaden their understanding of how societies grow and develop. Examples include partnering with the nutrition department to address malnutrition in a host country, or collaborating with the school of public health to design an HIV program (Riner & Becklenberg, 2001).

Choosing a location can be done in several different ways. It is best if you have ties or relationships with key personnel in the host country. This can help with logistics, translation, and networking, as well as student supervision. Collaboration is key. Partners in the host country can help with planning, and can be cultural brokers, helping bridge gaps between your own beliefs and culture and those of the host country (Jewell, 2007; Levi, 2009). Partners can be drawn from nongovernmental organizations (NGOs); professional organizations; other schools of nursing; other colleges; hospitals or clinics; charitable groups; government bodies; or any other appropriate group, whether local or international. When collaborating with any group, ensure your missions and visions are compatible in regard to humanitarian service, goals for the project, and student safety.

Since there are hundreds of NGOs, it is likely you can find an established program whose goals are similar enough to your own that a partnership will benefit both groups. Being able to work within an already established program is ideal because students can help facilitate the overall mission of the NGO, and once students leave, the work continues. For example, in Ecuador our students partner with a local NGO addressing malnutrition. Students help with growth and development screenings and teach health-related classes to local children. In return they have learned how the NGO works with local schools to improve nutrition by delivering soy milk and other fortified foods to the community. The NGO and our students gather data relevant to assessing the project's success collaboratively. Working with NGOs also offers an advantage in that the NGO can facilitate relationship building with key community players (Walton et al., 2004). In Ghana, we partner with an NGO that focuses on strengthening health care access in rural areas, providing opportunities for us to work in local clinics and schools. In some cases, collaborating with the NGO has helped to provide safe, clean housing in the area for our students.

Professional organizations in host countries can also be accommodating. One of our faculty met a nurse from Russia at a conference. This friendship led to an opportunity for our students to work with the Russian Nursing Organization (RNO) to provide teaching and interchange with nursing students. Although the language barrier seemed daunting, the RNO provided translators and a gateway into the Russian health care system. Students prepared their lessons before leaving, with input from the Russian group to ensure culture and beliefs were appropriately considered. The presentations were professionally translated to ensure the language was appropriate. In return, the Russian students taught our students about the Russian health care system.

Another way to work within a host country is to collaborate with a local school of nursing, as we did in Tonga. The partnership allowed our students to interact with local nursing students and partake in a wide variety of learning experiences set up by the school. Similarly, we partnered with a nursing school in Jordan. There, because of the language barrier, we arranged for Jordanian students who spoke English to "buddy" with our students. This partnership was especially successful in bridging cultural barriers.

In partnering with a school, be sure to discuss any possible fees that might be required. In addition, some countries, states, and even boards of nursing require that you submit paperwork proving your qualifications and statements of liability insurance. Going to work in a heath care facility because someone at the facility invited you without clearing it through professional organizations can lead to bad will and the inability to successfully complete your planned experience.

If you are not partnering with nursing schools in the host country, a significant consideration is how your proposed program might affect nursing programs there. It is important to contact local nursing schools to ensure you do not impact clinical learning options for their students. Going to the host country when school is not in session is one way to avoid this conflict. However, if you are there at the same time, arranging to buddy with local students in the clinical experience, as we did in Jordan, may be another option.

As you begin working in other countries, networking and word of mouth often lead to opportunities in other parts of the host country or in neighboring countries. While the idea of running two or more programs may seem daunting, with experience, your confidence in your ability to evaluate a potential site and set up a program grows. For example, after we established a site in Argentina with an NGO, another NGO contacted the college to ask if we would evaluate a hospital in Ecuador for a similar program. Our successful experience in Argentina, along with previous experience in Guatemala, meant that the college was willing to open another site. We sent two people to Ecuador to do the requested evaluation and plan for future experiences there with students. The Ecuador partnership is with a hospital oversight committee and has opened doors to additional partnerships with NGOs in Ecuador.

We have learned that developing more than a few relationships in the same area can dilute the student experience and the ability to give back to our hosts. Then again, multiple partners allow work in different parts of the country so that we do not outstay our welcome.

Planning Considerations

Once you have decided that you would like to establish a service-learning program in a particular location, a few guidelines will make the process easier. First, it is in the best interests of both parties to agree on expected time frames at the start of the relationship.

For example, the host may be interested in a short visit of a week or two or a lengthier visit of several weeks or months.

Communication is a significant consideration in traveling to a country where your own language is not spoken. Language differences and time zones, as well as differing cultural expectations related to the timeliness of responses, may complicate carrying out necessary arrangements during the planning stage. Once on-site, language and culture will likely continue to present challenges. Hiring translators, although expensive, may be necessary. It is vital all participants learn how to work professionally and responsibly with interpreters. Participants should not expect their hosts to understand English and should attempt to learn at least basic communication in the host language, such as greetings and giving thanks.

If students are developing materials for the host community, they should apply the principles of health literacy to ensure that recipients will be able to understand the terminology used (U.S. Department of Health and Human Services [HHS], 2010; Yu, 2005). Students fluent in the host language are the only students who should assist in translating written materials; however, even they must be cautioned about misunderstanding of cultural nuances, and therefore, should have all work reviewed by native speakers who are residents of the host country. It is preferable to have material professionally translated for the host country before arrival. This helps decrease misunderstandings and miscommunications, and teaches students the importance of following the standards outlined in the National Standards on Culturally and Linguistically Appropriate Services (HHS, 2001). The use of pictures and white space is important, but these should be culturally appropriate.

Overcoming our ethnocentric ideas is a challenge for everyone, and is especially critical to gaining an appreciation of the host country, especially if it is a less developed country. Students may see their experience as a mission to be "saviors" rather than to learn what the host country has to offer. Certainly, one goal of the project is for students to share their nursing knowledge and experiences, but another is to identify the strengths and abilities of the hosts and build a partnership. Students need time and opportunities to interact with health care teams in the host country to recognize what they can learn from others. Having the students keep journals or complete reflective writing assignments may help them process their feelings and thoughts about the experience and, over time, will help mold their attitudes toward and understanding of their purpose in the service-learning project. It is appreciation that opens doors to collaboration.

Host Country Perspectives

After identifying partners within the host country, it is critical to ensure that everyone understands the goals and purposes of the partnership. The relationship should be balanced and reciprocal. A planning meeting to delineate goals and establish intended outcomes should take place prior to bringing students abroad. A few simple goals with minimal steps are less likely to cause confusion due to language, as small variances in word use can cause misinterpretations. A mid-way meeting is helpful to determine if the experience is on track, with a final evaluation meeting at the end to discuss how things went and the potential for further visits.

Assessing what the host community would like from a service-learning program is not always easy. The host community may not be certain of their goals and may be hesitant to ask for particular services for fear of causing embarrassment if the service cannot be provided. In addition, the host is likely knowledgeable about health concerns or gaps in care, but may not be sure of the best way to address those concerns. When working in countries with economic difficulties, it is likely that even the best trained providers at the most prestigious institutions may have minimal or no access to literature databases that could help them solve their problems. In several cases, we have used our database resources to find data pertinent to partners' concerns so they can review the literature and make protocol decisions. As needed, we help with translation. This has led to some significant changes in care and outcomes. For example, if the collaboration is long term and you are desirous to change nursing practices some providers in the host country can be appointed as adjunct faculty allowing them to have access to data bases. In our experience, several host communities have first asked for an assessment of their situation. This is a great way to begin a balanced partnership as you work together to better understand their concerns and their system. Community-driven projects are the most successful and sustainable projects (Ailenger, Molloy, & Sacasa, 2009; Bently & Ellison, 2007; Unite for Sight, 2010-2011). This basic principle of public health nursing is critical for the future of the relationship (Bosworth et al., 2006; DeCamp, 2007; Levi, 2009). Assessing and understanding current resources and what is working helps build the partnership and creates strong bonds.

When the host community has not been forthcoming with ideas, we have found it helpful to ask questions about their patients, workflow, and even their health care philosophy as we walk through the facility. This can spark conversations that lead to a project valuable to the host. For instance, a simple question about prenatal care in Argentina led to the hosts asking that we survey women about why they seek or do not seek prenatal care. As we worked together, trust was gained and more information was shared.

Importantly, those who have invited you may have a different vision than those with whom you will actually be working. Building relationships of trust at all levels is critical if buy-in and openness are to permeate the partnership. It cannot be just the leaders who want you to come; people on the front line also need buy in or there may be resistance to change. This can be done by being open and asking for assistance from front-line personnel in the preparation and, especially, presentation of training sessions (Levi, 2009; Morgan, 2007).

Having the same faculty members return to the site regularly also helps build trust in the partnership. When we are accepted as peers, our insights and suggestions are more likely to be easily accepted. In our experience, asking for feedback and suggestions along the way has also helped build trusted partnerships.

The needs of the host nursing community can be categorized into three themes. These are nursing education, nursing resources, and nursing cultural exchanges.

Nursing Education

Prior to identifying the educational needs of the host site, it is vital that you understand the role of the nurse in health care and the context in which nurses work in the host country. Not understanding the political and social history of a country is a pitfall that can lead to not being accepted and issues with safety (Unite for Sight, 2010-11). The terminology to describe nurses, their role, and their education differs greatly among countries and even facilities in the same country (Critchley et al., 2009). This is not just in regard to the education required to be a nurse, but in the role and value assigned to nursing. Most host communities that want to partner with us see the role of the nurse as poorly defined or as needing to change but are unsure of what needs to be done and how to do it. For example, the nurses we worked with in Argentina were on government contracts for their hours, and there was no provision of time for handoff. The nurses were aware this situation was dangerous but did not know what to do about it. Through dialogue with nurses and management, we helped the facility implement a handoff protocol, and the situation improved.

It is critical to learn as much as possible about the culture and health care system of the host country, as this will impact what you teach and how you interact (Ailinger et al., 2009; DeCamp, 2007; Eyler, 2002). Understanding beliefs of the host country related to the cultural expectations of men and women; the organization of health care; the ratio of medical doctors to nurses; and the role of providers, families, and others in maintaining health and treating illness are all important.

Sometimes the host country may want to adopt a new model of nursing, a project which is much more difficult than teaching nursing care. Unfortunately, the philosophical approach to nursing in one country cannot be simply transplanted into another. Attempting to do this may create an unbalanced relationship – essentially, doing as the Victorians did and "conquering others" rather than partnering with them (DeCamp, 2007; Harrison & Malone, 2004). For example, many duties carried out by nurses in the U.S. are performed in Tonga with great reverence by family members. Trying to change this would be offensive to the families, patients, and community. Even when teaching specific techniques such as neonatal resuscitation, we have learned the importance of understanding the resources available in the host community, and adapting the training as appropriate. For example, teaching about oxygen administration when no oxygen is likely to be available is not helpful.

Assessment of needs in the host community is an ongoing process, and students benefit greatly from the process. By researching the host country prior to setting out – that is, its health care system, government, educational system, and culture – students come to understand differences and similarities between the host country and their own (Crigger, Brannigan, & Baird, 2006; DeCamp, 2007; Kirkham, Van Hofwegen, & Pankratz, 2009; Levi, 2009), and can prepare evidence-based, culturally appropriate teaching modules related to topics of concern. Potential topics are limitless, but may include HIV/AIDS prevention, hygiene, sanitation, infectious disease, chronic disease management, nutrition, or first aid, among others.

Key to success is frequent meetings to evaluate the program's content as well as how well it is functioning. In Argentina, our exchanges began as faculty-to-faculty training, but working closely with the nurse manager and the nurses allowed the group to identify other projects and needs. Here, observation is the best teacher. Seeing the work of nurses from the host country shows our students a lot about caring for patients with low resources, while the role modeling of our students exposes their nurses to other ways of approaching their patients.

For example, in Argentina we were invited to teach the nurses we worked with about our knowledge of the role of nursing in childbirth, developmental care, and feeding in the neonatal intensive care unit (NICU). Traditionally, nurses in Argentina (and in many developing countries) do not provide support to women in labor. Medical residents monitor the women for progress but do little, if any, labor support. Our faculty members offered training on U.S. practices related to the role of the nurse in supporting labor. Following this, our students were accepted into the clinical setting, where they gained valuable experience while modeling how nurses could help women during childbirth. Years later, when the hospital was renovated, the rooms were designed to allow for labor support by nurses and doulas (trained labor support specialists). Similarly, we noted that many babies in the NICU were not developing correctly due to their positioning, and mothers were not encouraged to hold and interact with their infants. Our students, along with our nursing faculty, were able to provide in-service training in both developmental and kangaroo care. The mothers reported that taking part in their infant's care and development helped them feel closer to their babies. After several years, the trust level with both doctors and nurses was such that we were able to work with them to develop and implement an evidence-based feeding protocol for preterm infants, which made a significant difference in the infants' outcomes.

Nursing Resources

Another area where host countries may want assistance is efficient use of material resources and equipment. They may also want help with a critically low supply of nursing manpower.

Developing countries have limited resources. In many countries, care providers may reuse gauze and other equipment or may not have adequate gloves, blankets, and basic supplies. You should plan to bring adequate supplies for your cohort so you do not deplete their already meager stores. Although it may be appropriate to bring some provisions for the host community when participating in service-learning opportunities, it is important to not encourage your hosts to become dependent on gifted supplies. This is an easy trap to fall into because the host community may identify materials as their biggest need. Yet bringing supplies and equipment without first building a relationship may make the relationship that develops lopsided rather than equal. It may be best to start with supplies that students will be using when in the host country, and leaving any "extras" when the students return home.

Knowledge is a resource that may be needed but is not always identified. As nursing schools, our greatest resource is the knowledge that we can impart. It is for this reason we try to focus on providing education, not provisions. We have found it helpful to say something like, "We do not have a lot of financial resources, but we will willingly share our time and our knowledge."

A further resource for the host country may be manpower. Often, host countries have concerns or needs but not the resources to fully identify either the root cause or the extent of an issue. Students can provide the temporary manpower needed to assess the situation and identify potential solutions. For example, malnutrition is a concern in a variety of the host countries we have worked with, particularly Ecuador and Argentina. Our partners in each host country knew malnutrition was an issue, but were not sure of the extent and severity of the problem. In this regard, collaborative data collection has worked well. Nursing students worked alongside local community volunteers to perform basic screenings, and were also able to interview parents and observe family meals to determine what was lacking. Along with training volunteers in the host country in data collection methods, we were able to ensure the data was given back to the community. Together, we developed ideas and recommendations for what could be done next.

Nursing Cultural Exchanges

The final major request that many host countries have is cultural exchanges. Whether or not these countries have the resources and educational opportunities typical in the United States, they realize that learning from other systems and cultures enhances their skills and abilities (Bosworth et al., 2006; Lange & Ailinger, 2001; Riner & Becklenberg, 2001). We have learned that such cultural exchanges can broaden our own minds as well. This is why we try to offer one or two service-learning opportunities in developed countries along with those in less-developed nations. For example, we have partnered with a large medical hospital in Taiwan. This hospital has much of the same advanced technology as hospitals in the United States, while also practicing traditional healing methods such as cupping, coining, and acupuncture. Our students are partnered with nurses in the hospital, as well as nurses working in the community. The students are able to help in education and basic nursing functions, while at the same time learning about a different health care system and cultural practices.

The challenge is always ensuring that we address the needs of the host country and not only our own priorities. As outsiders we may see concerns that we think are top priority, but we must remember the host community may view other needs as more urgent. Working in partnerships is important as students learn, so that when they become nursing leaders they are able to practice in a culturally sensitive manner.

Program Evaluation

Program evaluation is critical. To be complete, the evaluation should be based on the perceptions of the students and faculty, the host partner, and the local people.

Host Site Perspective

To evaluate the program from the perspective of the host site, an effective method is to conduct qualitative interviews with the partner in the host country and people with whom you interacted. Questions can be designed to elicit information such as: (1) Did we meet the needs of the host site? (2) What were the positive aspects of having the students present? (3) What could be done better in the future? (4) Were there any negative effects of the interaction? Ideally, a person not connected with the project should conduct the interviews, and should do so at a time when students and faculty are not present, as their presence may bias responses. In some areas this may be difficult due to time differences or a lack of communication tools (telephones or internet).

When evaluating the impact on the host country, it is important to assess whether the host country partners are becoming too dependent on the project. This may be the case if the host partners seem to be demanding or expecting too much in the way of supplies and material goods.

Student and Faculty Perspective

Interviews and reflective writings can both be used to assess students' experiences. Questions to ask students include: (1) What was the aspect of the experience that impacted you the most? (2) How did the experience affect your nursing skills and professional plans? (3) How did the experience influence your desire to serve in the future?

Depending on the goal, purpose, and length of the service-learning experience, quantitative tools may also prove helpful in evaluating the program. The focus of our programs is not just enhancing our students' nursing skills and knowledge, but also helping them become more culturally aware. Many tools can be used to help assess cultural competence or awareness. Some are specific to nursing (Caffrey, 2005; Campinha-Bacote, 2003; Jeffries, 2006; Rew, Becker, Cookston, Khosropour, & Martinez, 2003; Zorn, 1998). Other tools that are not specific to nursing may also be appropriate; tools designed to measure cultural competence, a global perspective, self-efficacy, or altruism have been developed by scholars in other disciplines (Allen, 2009; Braskamp, Braskamp, Merrill, & Engberg, 2010; Fantini, 2006; Hughes & Hood, 2007; Paige, 2004). The best tool to use depends upon the purpose and intended learning outcomes of the experience. Many of these tools are often best used as pre- and posttest measures, but service-learning experiences need to be a sufficient length if these tools are to be used in a pre-/posttest capacity.

With all the work involved in setting up a service-learning experience, it is critical to evaluate its effectiveness for all parties. The key concept of service-learning is a reciprocal relationship where both host countries and nursing schools benefit.

Case Study: Ecuador

Our Ecuador GSL experience is one of the longest-running global service-learning programs in the Brigham Young University College of Nursing. The genesis of the program goes back to 2000, when an NGO approached our college to ask for help with four large welfare hospitals they were running in the city. The hospitals included a 900+ bed general hospital, a maternity hospital that averages over 125 births a day, a pediatric hospital, and a psychiatric hospital. The hospitals' administrators were cognizant of the challenges they faced, but since these were welfare-based hospitals supported by local donations, they did not have adequate resources to provide the care they wanted to. The NGO asked us to conduct a survey in order to identify the most critical problem areas, and to offer suggestions for how the care and service provided could be improved.

A faculty member and a friend of the nursing college (a pediatric nurse) made an initial visit to see the hospitals and to meet with many of the administrators. The evaluators assessed areas of concern and wrote a report. One immediate action was to make changes to the frequent rotation of nurses between units, which made it difficult for nurses to become expert in any one area. The report also identified continuing education as a problem, especially given the hospitals' shortage of nursing staff. The report discussed ways by which the college could help the hospitals structure in continuing education classes in key areas.

At the time, we had two Spanish-speaking programs keeping us busy, so it was not until 2004 that we were able to focus on Ecuador. At that point, we developed a plan with emphasis on continuing education among the nursing staff to address areas of major concern in patient care: infection control, basic and advanced life support, and basic skills. It was agreed that a group of our graduate-level nursing students would travel to Ecuador for a three-week program of teaching at two of the hospitals. The students would receive partial credit for their chronic disease course for participation in the Ecuador project. In May of 2004, a group of eight nursing students arrived in Ecuador with two college of nursing faculty members, bringing prepared lesson plans with them.

Once the group arrived, in the initial meeting with the hospital administrators, it was discovered our expectations and those of the host country differed. The administrators were expecting continuous classes for about 50 nurses over the course of the few weeks, while we were prepared to give a few classes over and over again to many nurses. Thus, a lot of quick preparation was needed, and our students put in many late nights as they prepared for the next day's teaching. We learned that communication between the home and host institution is vital, but language barriers are real. Both institutions had thought they fully understood the other. We learned flexibility is the key ingredient to make an international collaboration work.

In looking back at the first year, we noted that initially, most of the collaboration focused on addressing the needs of the host community. There was little communication about our students' need to meet objectives for their courses. Objectives for the students were discussed during the experience and were met in roundabout ways. After the first year, it was clear there would need to be more give and take in everybody's expectations.

Perceptions about logistics were also an interesting challenge. The hospital administration was highly concerned about the health and safety of the group. They had prepared housing in the hospital for the students, along with meals in the cafeteria. This allowed our hosts to feel comfortable about our general well being. They even provided security day and night in front of our rooms, as well as western food (pancakes with maple syrup). Their goal was to keep us safe and protected from the "outside world."

This was a challenge for us, as one of our goals was to expose our students to a different culture. We felt this included living among the people, eating their food, and experiencing their surroundings. However, we appreciated the feelings of our hosts. Again, we learned that we needed to be clear in our communication without being insensitive. We were able to express our desires to be more exposed to the culture over the following years. We told our hosts respectfully that though we appreciated the offer of housing within the hospital, we felt living downtown and eating local food better met our needs.

A happy compromise was met when the administration suggested a nearby hotel that was safe but culturally appropriate. Our hosts still feel the need to provide security at the airport when we arrive and when we leave the country, and at other larger events. We appreciate their efforts and concern for our safety. Sometimes the students do not understand the burden of responsibility that is felt by the host country, and this provides an eloquent teaching moment in our Ecuador experience.

During our first year, the host community was caught off guard by the need felt by our students to stay in frequent connection through email or phone to their loved ones at home. One computer with internet access had been provided for 16 people. This was a major issue for the students, some of whom were engaged or newly married. We were able to "fix" the situation by assigning computer time so all students had equal access. This was a challenge we had not anticipated, and it became a learning experience for both our hosts and ourselves. Now, when sending students on a service-learning experience we plan for this need.

Even with the success of the first year behind us, we faced a challenge in setting the course for future years. We wanted to help our hosts, but we didn't want to *be* the help. We wanted to teach them to teach themselves, and we wondered if the successful precedent we had set was unsustainable. Moreover, while the first group sent to Ecuador comprised graduate-level nursing students, our plans called for future cohorts to be undergraduates – inexperienced in nursing, let alone teaching. It was obvious we needed to communicate this change to our Ecuadorian partners, and ask how we could meet the needs of both parties.

Fortunately, over the years we have been able to meld the desires and needs of both organizations. We have been able to take a few graduate nursing students, along with our undergraduate cohort, to continue training small groups of nurses in the hospitals; the nurses trained then go on to become teachers for their colleagues. Meanwhile, our undergraduate students have the opportunity to work alongside Ecuadorian nurses in the hospitals and provide care to patients. (The numbers of undergraduate and graduate students have varied through the years.) Overall, we are better about communicating what we are able to provide and what we want to learn.

For our part, we have learned more about what the Ecuadorians expect from us in terms of the classes we teach. They feel pride in completing the classes, and they were surprised that we had not thought about graduation certificates or a concluding ceremony. This was promptly rectified in the program's second year: we had certificates made, with the appropriate signatures and seals, and arranged a well-thought-out concluding ceremony. The Ecuadorians are also meticulous record keepers with regard to attendance, and this has made it easier to track participants over the years. We have been able to conduct a few research projects on the effect of the teaching that has taken place.

Our partners in Ecuador usually organize exit interviews. Our students are always honored to be guests of the hospital's top administration and to have their voices heard. Using information from these interviews, we have been able to review the GSL experience of our students, as well as assess the progress of the hospitals. We greatly appreciate how our Ecuadorian hosts have felt it necessary to complete each program in this way. They are very interested in how the students view their experience; in turn, we feel valued and are able to express our appreciation for the host country and all they do for us.

References

Ailinger, R. L., Molloy, S. B., & Sacasa, E. R. (2009). Community health nursing student experience in Nicaragua. *Journal of Community Health Nursing, 26,* 47–53. doi: 1080/07370010902805072

Allen, J. (2010). Improving cross-cultural care and antiracism in nursing education: A literature review. *Nurse Education Today, 30*(4), 314-20. doi: 10.1016/j.nedt2009.08.007

Bailey, P., Carpenter, D., & Harrington, P. (Eds.). (1999). *Integrating community service into nursing education: A guide to service learning.* New York: Springer Publishing Company.

Bently, R., & Ellison, K. (2007). Increasing cultural competence in nursing through international service-learning. *Nurse Educator, 32*(5), 2007–2011. doi:10.1097/01. NNE.0000289385.14007.b4

Bosworth, T. L., Haloburdo, E. P., Hetrick, C., Patchett, K., Thompson, M. A., & Welch, M. (2006). International partnerships to promote quality care: Faculty groundwork, student projects, and outcomes. *The Journal of Continuing Education in Nursing, 37*(1), 32–38.

Braskamp, L. A., Braskamp, D. C. , Merrill, K. C., & Engberg, M. E. (2010). *Global perspective inventory (GPI).* http:gpi.central.edu.

Caffrey, R. A. (2005). Improving the cultural competence of nursing students: Results of integrating cultural content in the curriculum and international immersion experience. *Journal of Nursing Education, 44*(5), 234–240.

Campinha-Bacote, J. (2003). *The process of cultural competence in the delivery of healthcare services: A culturally competent model of care* (4th ed.). Cincinnati, OH: Transcultural C.A.R.E. Associates.

Crigger M. J., Brannigan, M., & Baird, M. (2006). Compassionate nursing professionals as good citizens of the world. *Advances in Nursing Science, 29*(1), 15–26.

Critchley, K. A., Richardson, E., Aarts, C., Campbell, B., Hemmingway, A., Koskinen, L., ... Nordstrom, P. (2009). Student experiences with an international public health exchange project. *Nurse Educator, 34*(2), 69–74. doi:10.1097/ NNE.0b013e3181990ed4.

DeCamp, M. (2007). Scrutinizing global short-term medical outreach. *Hastings Center Report, 37*(6), 21–23.

Eyler, J. (2002). Reflecting on service: Helping nursing students get the most from service-learning. *Journal of Nursing Education, 41*(10), 453–456.

Fantini, A. E. (2006). *Assessment tools of intercultural communicative competence.* Retrieved from http://www.experiment.org/documents/AppendixF.pdf

Harrison, L., & Malone, K. (2004). A study abroad experience in Guatemala: Learning first-hand about health, education and social welfare in a low-resource country. *International Journal of Nursing Education Scholarship, 1*(1), 1–15.

Hughes, K. H., & Hood, L. J. (2007). Teaching methods and an outcome tool for measuring cultural sensitivity in undergraduate nursing students. *Journal of Transcultural Nursing, 18*(1), 57–62.

Jeffries, M. R. (2006). *Teaching cultural competence in nursing and health care: Inquiry, action and innovation.* New York: Springer Publishing Co.

Jewell, G. (2007). Contextual empowerment: The impact of health brigade involvement on the women of Miratior, Nicaragua. *Journal of Transcultural Nursing,18*(1), 49–56.

Kirkham, S., Van Hofwegen, L., & Pankratz, D. (2009). Keeping vision: Sustaining social consciousness with nursing students following international learning experiences. *International Journal of Nursing Education Scholarship, 6*(1), 1–15.

Lange, I., & Ailinger, R. L. (2001). International nursing faculty exchange model: A Chile-USA case. *International Nursing Review, 48,* 109–116.

Levi, A. (2009). The ethics of nursing student international clinical experiences. *Journal of Obstetric, Gynecologic, and Neonatal Nursing, 38*(1), 94–99. doi: 10.1111/j.1552-6909.2008.0031.x.

Morgan, M. (2007). Another view of "humanitarian ventures" and "fistula tourism." *International Urogynecology Journal, 18,* 705–707.

Paige, R. M. (2004). Instrumentation in intercultural training. In D. Landis, J. Bennett, & M. J. Bennett (Eds.), *Handbook of intercultural training* (3rd ed.) (pp. 85 –127). Thousand Oaks, CA: Sage Publications.

Rew, L., Becker, H., Cookston, J., Khosropour, S., & Martinez, S. (2003). Measuring cultural awareness in nursing students. *Journal of Nursing Education, 42*(6), 249–257.

Riner, M. E., & Becklenberg, A. (2001). Partnering with a sister city for an international service- learning experience. *Journal of Transcultural Nursing, 12*(3), 234–240.

United States Department of Health and Human Services, Office of Disease Prevention and Health Promotion. (2010). *National action plan to improve health literacy.* Washington, DC: Author.

United States Department of Health and Human Services, Office of Minority Health. (2001). *National standards for culturally and linguistically appropriate services in health care.* Washington, DC: Author.

Unite for Sight (2010-2011). Pitfalls in global health work. Retrieved March 31, 2011, from http://www.uniteforsight.org/pitfalls-in-development/pitfalls-in-global-health#_ftn9

Walton, D. A., Farmer, P. E., Lambert, W., Léandre, F., Koenig, S. P., & Mukherjee, J. S. (2004). Integrated HIV prevention and care strengthens primary health care: Lessons from rural Haiti. *Journal of Public Health Policy, 25,* 137–158.

Yu, M. (2005). Sociolinguistic competence in the complimenting act of native Chinese and American English speakers: A mirror of cultural value. *Language and Speech, 48*(1), 91–119.

Zorn, C.R. (1996). The long-term impact on nursing students participating in international education. *Journal of Professional Nursing, 12*(2), 106-110.

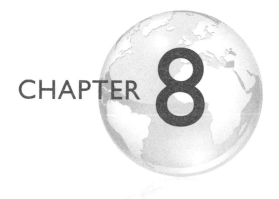

CHAPTER 8

Nursing Students as Program Partners

Donna M. (Costello) Nickitas

Global service-learning (GSL) is a form of experiential learning that is fast becoming a core component of nursing education. GSL brings students from the classroom into the community to collaborate with diverse stakeholders on an organized service activity to address real health or social problems. GSL models bridge classroom theory with active learning in the community and use the world to impart to students knowledge and skills that are related to course content.

Experiencing the "real world" through GSL engages students in an exchange of ideas with people from different communities and cultures, and enhances their sense of civic and social responsibility (Bringle & Hatcher, 1995; Grusky, 2000; Kiely, 2005; Monard-Weissman, 2003a, 2003b).

In short, GSL uses a local lens to ignite students' interest and capacity as global citizens – as people who can make a difference. The strategy is well suited for nursing education because it offers students context-specific opportunities to practice core skills; to gain new skills specific to community-based nursing, such as community assessment and health promotion skills; and to develop cultural competence and a sense of social responsibility – all while delivering much-needed nursing and health care services to underserved populations (Seifer & Calleson, 2004; Reising et al., 2008; Witchger-Hansen et al., 2007).

Nursing Students as Program Partners in Global Service-Learning

From the very beginning, nursing students must be active and engaged partners in the GSL experience. To accomplish this, students should be included from the early stages in creating campus-community agreements designed to fill a health care need. As they help develop and negotiate service-learning agreements, student come to understand the real nature of the service need and how best to address it. They learn to consider the following questions:

- Is the service to be provided useful, and does it address needs, concerns, and issues identified by nursing students as well as other stakeholders?

- Does the service consider both students' learning objectives and stakeholders' knowledge and assets? Does the service build capacity for civic engagement and global citizenry?

- Do faculty, students, and community partners recognize that most health issues and problems may not be solved in the allotted time, for example, in one semester or less?

- Do students and community partners have realistic expectations about the short and long-term goals of a global service-learning project? Does the project present opportunities for sustainable service-learning work now and in the future?

Building Global Partnerships

Global partnerships are the means by which the commitment to global health in nursing education programs can reach beyond the classroom. Research has shown the importance of equality between the academic institution and the community partner in planning educational experiences that meet community needs while fostering meaningful and explicit learning for students (Nokes, Nickitas, Keida, & Neville, 2005; Riley, Beal, & Lancaster, 2008). Table 8-1 presents the Principles of Good Community-Campus Partnerships established by Community-Campus Partnerships for Health (CCPH), a nonprofit organization that promotes health, broadly defined, through partnerships between communities and institutions of higher education (CCPH, 2011).

Table 8-1. Principles of Good Community-Campus Partnerships

Adopted by the CCPH board of directors, October 2006

1. Partnerships form to serve a specific purpose and may take on new goals over time.

2. Partners have agreed upon mission, values, goals, measurable outcomes and accountability for the partnership.

3. The relationship between partners is characterized by mutual trust, respect, genuineness, and commitment.

4. The partnership builds upon identified strengths and assets, but also works to address needs and increase capacity of all partners.

5. The partnership balances power among partners and enables resources among partners to be shared.

6. Partners make clear and open communication an ongoing priority by striving to understand each other's needs and self-interests, and developing a common language.

7. Principles and processes for the partnership are established with the input and agreement of all partners, especially for decision-making and conflict resolution.

8. There is feedback among all stakeholders in the partnership, with the goal of continuously improving the partnership and its outcomes.

9. Partners share the benefits of the partnership's accomplishments.

10. Partnerships can dissolve and need to plan a process for closure.

Creating global partnerships that are both meaningful and sustainable requires that nursing students and community partners invest time in getting to know one another, working together, and learning to trust one another. This relationship-building process involves compromise and negotiation, and acceptance of one another's strengths and weaknesses. All partners must be patient when mistakes occur and take time to thank each other for each one's service and commitment.

Successful partnerships typically have a clear format, structure, and scope, and reasonable agreed-upon expected outcomes. Before negotiating global partnerships, consider the following:

- How much time will the partnership require? What human and financial resources will be available from the campus and the community? What expenses and costs will be incurred by the service? Consider the boundaries of time, place, participants, and resources.

- How will services be delivered and outcomes shared and acknowledged?

- Is there a written partnership agreement or contract? Who are the key stakeholders for such an agreement?

Bringing nursing students to the table and teaching them how to build global partnerships is crucial. They must be a part of the discussion and help define the criteria of what constitutes a sound and reasonable partnership

Nursing Students as Effective Team Members and Partners

Before people can build trust and relationships with external partners, they must first build trust among themselves. That is, they must become an effective team. A team, as defined by Katzenbach and Smith (1993), is a small number of people with complementary skills who are committed to a common purpose, performance goals, and approach for which they are mutually accountable. Reaching that stage of common approach and mutual accountability is not always easy. When working with nursing students to build a GSL partnership, faculty members must take the time to discuss and demonstrate how effective teams are developed. Students need support in learning how to function within a team, and how team members clarify roles and responsibilities, create space for members to experience and process error, and build trust. As they guide students through this process, faculty members must recognize that all students enter a team with their own unique characteristics, experiences, and approaches to learning and to teamwork.

In the global service-learning context, the students first must learn to see one another's perspectives, attitudes, and interests as well as to assess their competence, abilities, and shared values as they relate to the team. Beyond that, students must recognize that different cultures shape trust differently, and that cultural differences do exist when campus-community partnerships are formed.

Once students become familiar with how effective teams are managed and how partnerships are formed, they can ponder the following questions to nurture effective teamwork:

- Does my team share my values and goals?

- Does my team have the requisite knowledge, ability, and skills for the project it will be embarking on?

- Will my team honor its commitments to the community partners?

- Will my team tell me what I need to know?

- Does my team want me to succeed? If so, how?

Faculty members must be patient as they guide students through the team building process. They must monitor, support, and evaluate the process as students agree upon the type of shared leadership they need to guide their service-learning experience. Each student must understand his or her role not only in the team but also within the total partnership, and align that role with those of the community partner(s). Partnership skills are best fostered when there is balance and impartial thinking. No student should feel isolated or disrespected because of a different viewpoint. In the beginning, faculty must be diligent about maintaining a safe forum for the open sharing of ideas, concerns, and conflicts. Efforts should be made to help all partners acquire the appropriate roles and responsibilities as they:

- Develop a set of agreements and operating principles to guide the interaction and work of the partnership.

- Draft a mission statement and define core values about the global service-learning experience.

- Reflect, assess, evaluate, and make adjustments and refinements as needed for the partnership.

- Set reasonable expectations about partners' roles and the performance of the partnership.

Applying Learning in Meaningful Ways Through Reflection

Global service-learning involves more than students learning about the daily realities of life in another community or country and becoming familiar with another culture. It creates collaborative opportunities that have the potential to provide insights into historical, social, cultural, economic, and political experiences of the host community. These collaborative activities may foster greater student commitment towards social action, civic engagement, and meaningful global citizenship. To build civic and social responsibility within the profession, nursing students must be exposed to these responsibilities in their formative education. Students must understand how the core values of nursing – individual responsibility, autonomy, and altruism – impact nursing care, and how to act on these values throughout their professional careers (Kelley & Joel, 1995; Kenney, 1996; Rutty, 1998).

Watson (2008) suggests that competent, caring professional nurses are the most precious resource of the current U.S. health care system. To retain that resource, a new generation of health professionals must ensure caring and healing for the public, while learning about the value of serving others. Thus, nurse faculty can foster civic and social responsibility in undergraduate nursing students by developing service activities that seek to serve the broader society (Boutain, 2008). Service-learning thus may contribute to a student's acquisition of knowledge and skills that are integral to the nurse's professional identity and practice (Riley & Beal, 2010).

To ensure meaningful learning from a global service-learning experience, participating students should engage in structured reflection, whether orally – for instance, through group dialogue – or in written form, through journals and other assignments (Kiely, 2005; Kiely, Kiely, & Hartman, 2005). Journals can be written either in a hardcopy notebook, or in an online journal format by the individual or collectively as a group experience. Reflection and dialogue facilitate intellectual, emotional, and social processing of service-learning experiences (Kiely, 2005), and it is through them that students develop a sense of social responsibility, advocacy, active citizenship, intellectual growth, and critical thinking. Reflection also helps to prevent the development or reinforcement of prejudices and false assumptions about those in the community being served, and helps students feel more comfortable working with people who are different from themselves (Bentley & Ellison, 2005; Eyler 2002; Kiely, 2004).

Case Study: The Woza Moya Project

Since 2001, the Hunter-Bellevue School of Nursing at Hunter College, a large public university located in the heart of New York City, has integrated service-learning into its undergraduate curriculum. Nursing students enrolled in the introductory nursing course learn about the concepts and principles of service-learning and participate in service-learning projects during their first academic semester. In our first global service-learning experience, launched in 2009, our students partnered with a community in South Africa, well beyond their geographic boundaries. However, our students never left the country. Rather, they built a virtual global partnership.

Woza Moya is a nongovernmental organization (NGO) that provides care and support for people affected by HIV and AIDS in the Ofafa Valley, located near KwaZulu-Natal, South Africa. The Woza Moya Project was born in April 2000 as a community-based and -owned project in response to the devastating impact of AIDS in the region. Woza Moya provides ongoing services to orphans and vulnerable children, home-based care, HIV and AIDS information and counseling, food security, basic medicines, and paralegal and advocacy services. The project is now firmly established and widely respected not only within the local communities, but among the network of NGOs in KwaZulu and within South Africa as a whole. It is considered a "model response" to the tragedy of AIDS in Africa

In 2009, I invited a Hunter-Bellevue colleague, Dr. Kathleen Nokes, to help establish a service-learning project involving Woza Moya. Dr. Nokes had a longstanding relationship with nurses at Woza Moya, and agreed to help facilitate the project. Without ever leaving our home campus, we built a partnership without walls, whereby we connect globally through Skype and the World Wide Web to the Woza Moya community.

The overall goal of the service-learning project became fundraising. As one student put it, "We wanted to raise as much money as possible to help Woza Moya obtain the necessary supplies needed to provide direct services." The students quickly realized that sending equipment and supplies overseas would be too costly, so they strategically and creatively managed a team of 18 to raise not only money, but awareness about the HIV/AIDS epidemic in South Africa and Woza Moya.

Within a 15-week semester, the students raised over $3,100 through campus bake sales, T-shirt sales, Facebook/PayPal donations, a faculty lunch, and contributions from friends and family. To date, the Hunter-Bellevue School of Nursing has contributed over $4,000 to Woza Moya. The Facebook page launched by the students (www.facebook.com/HunterforWozaMoya) has helped raise awareness and educate the Hunter College community about Woza Moya, serving as both an effective fundraising tool and a place to post relevant facts, articles, and videos on the project and the community. (Our 2010 service-learning project can be found on YouTube: HBSON NURS200 Woza Moya Presentation Fall 2010 at http://www.youtube.com/watch?v=QDKo3OxjtVU.)

Although the students were not able to physically care for the Woza Moya community, they felt every bit connected to them. Through effective teamwork, care and compassion, these students learned the core nursing values of human dignity, altruism, and integrity. They reached out via Skype, phone and email to the Woza Moya founder, Sue Hedden, and to the leaders of two U.S.-based organizations that support Woza Moya – Catherine Anderson of Ubuntu Charlotte, a charity based in Charlotte, South Carolina, and Kathy Cook, director of the South Coast Foundation, a private foundation that operates a grantmaking program in South Africa. The students came to recognize how nonprofit agencies are managed and supported.

Despite not having their "feet on the ground in South Africa," the students came to understand, appreciate, and support the mission of the Woza Moya Project. Suddenly, their fundraising activities, education and awareness campaign, and social networking had removed the geographic boundaries. The global partnership between the School of Nursing and Woza Moya turned out to be a meaningful global service-learning experience for the students and had a huge financial outcome for the project. Our students achieved a global service-learning experience without ever having to pack a bag or leave the country.

References

Boutain, D. M. (2008). Social justice as a framework for undergraduate community health clinical experiences in the United States. *International Journal of Nursing Education Scholarship, 5,* 1–12.

Bentley, R. and Ellison, K.J.(2005).Impact of a service learning project on nursing students. *Nursing Education Perspectives, 26*(5), 287-290.

Bringle, R., and Hatcher, J. A. (1995). Service learning curriculum for faculty. *The Michigan Journal of Community Service-Learning, 2,* 112–122.

Community-Campus Partnerships for Health. (2011) Principles of good community-campus partnerships. Retrieved from http://www.ccph.info/

Eyler, J. (2002) Reflecting on service: Helping nursing students get the most from service-learning. *Journal of Nursing Education, 4*(10), 453–456.

Grusky, S. (2000). International service learning: A critical guide from an impassioned advocate. *American Behavioral Scientist, 43*(5), 858–867.

Katzenbach, J. R., & Smith, D. K. (1993). *The wisdom of teams: Creating the high-performance organization.* Boston: Harvard Business School.

Kelley, L. Y., & Joel, L. (1995). *Dimensions of professional nursing.* New York: McGraw-Hill.

Kenney, J. (1996). *Philosophical and theoretical perspectives for advanced nursing practice.* Boston: Jones & Bartlett.

Kiely, R. (2004). A chameleon with a complex: Searching for transformation in international service learning. *Michigan Journal of Community Service Learning, 10*(2), 5–20.

Kiely, R. (2005). Transformative international service-learning. *Academic Exchange Quarterly, 9*(1), 275–281.

Kiely, R., Kiely, A., & Hartman, E. (2005). *International service-learning: What? Why? How?* Paper presented at the 57th Annual Conference of NAFSA: Association of International Educators, Seattle, WA.

Monard-Weissman, K. (2003a). Fostering a sense of social justice through international service-learning. *Academic Exchange Quarterly 7*(2), 164–169.

Monard-Weissman, K. (2003b). Enhancing caring capacities: A case study of an international service-learning program. *Journal of Higher Education Outreach and Engagement, 8*(2), 41–53.

Nokes, K., Nickitas, D., Keida, R., & Neville, S. (2005). Does service-learning increase cultural competency, critical thinking, and civic engagement? *Journal of Nursing Education, 44,* 65–70.

Reising, D. L., Shea, R. A., Allen, P. N., Laux, M. M., Hensel, D., & Watts, P. A. (2008). Using service-learning to develop health promotion and research skills in nursing students. *International Journal of Nursing Education Scholarship, 5,* 1–15.

Riley, J., &. Beal, J. (2010). Public service: Experienced nurses' views on social and civic responsibility. *Nursing Outlook 58*(3), 142–147.

Riley, J., Beal, J., & Lancaster, D. (2008). Scholarly nursing practice from the perspectives of experienced nurses. *Journal of Advanced Nursing, 61,* 425–435.

Rutty, J. (1998). The nature of philosophy of science, theory and knowledge relating to nursing and professionalism. *Journal of Advanced Nursing, 28,* 243–250.

Seifer, S. D., &. Calleson, D. C. (2004). Health professional faculty perspectives on community-based research: Implications for policy and practice. *Journal of Interprofessional Care, 18,* 416–427.

Watson, J. (2008). Social justice and human caring: A model of caring science as a hopeful paradigm for moral justice and humanity. *Creative Nursing, 14,* 54–61.

Witchger-Hansen, A. M., Muñoz, J., Crist, P. A., Gupta, J., Ideishi, R. I., Primeau, L. A., & Tupé, D. (2007). Service learning: Meaningful, community-centered professional skill development for occupational therapy students. *Occupational Therapy in Health Care, 21,* 25–49.

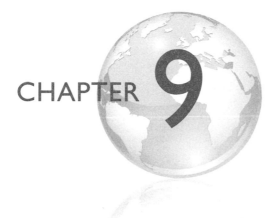

CHAPTER **9**

Exemplars of Global Service-Learning in Nursing

Cathleen M. Shultz
Freida Chavez
Amanda M. Giordano
Jane Sumner

Exemplar 1
An Early Holistic Service-Learning Program
Cathleen M. Shultz

From its inception in 1975, the Carr College of Nursing envisioned a nursing program in which students and faculty, through learning experiences, ministered to others with needs subtle or profound. The philosophy of the college was holistic, although the phrase "holistic" was not widely accepted at that time. Though the world of nursing outside the United States embraced "holistic care" more favorably, within the U.S. the idea was viewed with considerable skepticism except in rare conclaves of nursing education. In fact, U.S. state approval and national accreditation bodies believed that nursing should stick to the realms of the physical and psychological, and looked unkindly at any involvement of nurses in the spiritual beliefs and practices of others. Yet the roots of nursing education in the United States found many diploma programs teaching religious, faith-based and spiritual practices to help students understand and provide nursing care to diverse populations.

The Carr College of Nursing is part of the faith-based institution of Harding University, in Searcy, Arkansas; its mission statement is "Developing Nurses as Christian Servants." Searcy is a rural community about 50 miles northeast of Little Rock. In 1975, it had two small community hospitals, each with fewer than 100 beds. Harding's administration was determined to create a new baccalaureate nursing program in which holistic ministering as nurses would incubate and thrive – even in the dubious context of a national nursing education environment that was less than enthusiastic toward a holistic view of mankind. The Carr College faculty came from various regions of the United States and abroad. (The student body, to this day, comes from all states and well over 65 countries.) Their diversity of experiences, preparation and cultures joined with Harding's holistic philosophy to produce what, in time, would be known as global service-learning.

Building an educational initiative from scratch with minimal available printed resources or consultants for guidance requires long-term commitment and a refusal to be discouraged by setbacks. As we developed our first service-learning programs, we found that flexibility in scheduling, creativity, and mutual support are paramount. Under such circumstances, learning and teaching strategies perforce become experiential. At Harding, we saw that service-learning was holistic for all participants – the faculty, students, institution, and most important, the recipients of service learning. Service-learning created an environment of reciprocity among students, teachers, and recipients: one teaches one who teaches one who teaches one...and on the cycle continues. I am convinced that engagement in helping others is one of the most enriching of learning experiences, and service-learning can be life-changing for all involved. Certainly, I'm frequently amazed at the dramatic changes in knowledge, skills, attitudes, and behavior of learners and faculty as they prepare for, engage in, and reflect upon their service experiences.

Although numerous global service-learning opportunities abound, I specifically want to address a form that we call "health missions." Health mission service-learning, for Harding University nurses, has evolved into planned domestic and international programs that are organized by nursing faculty. Some health mission experiences are planned and taught solely by nursing faculty. Others, now the most predominant, are planned and taught in partnership with other departments at the university. After more than 35 years, we now have an international network of organizations, alumni, and supporters on whom we are inter- and intra-dependent.

At Harding, we believe in long-term commitment to our service-learning communities, and this belief underpins our health missions. We have four types of health mission programs. First, for over 35 years, we have regularly planned and implemented summer health mission programs in Africa, particularly Nigeria and Tanzania. Sites have rarely been changed, and then only because of imminent danger to student learners and faculty, such as the kidnappings for ransom so prevalent in Nigeria in recent years. Second, for over six years we have offered a semester abroad in Zambia, in partnership with the campus International Program Office. One advanced practice nursing faculty member prepares all students (from the nursing college and other departments) and travels with them on-site; other rotating university programs also send a faculty member. These programs predominantly involve care for AIDS orphans and nutrition programs in villages. Diarrhea and infectious diseases devastate the areas, and our participants learn to implement cost-effective and life-sustaining practices, such as rehydration. Third are domestic programs, with key efforts in initiating and staffing freestanding clinics that incorporate holistic care to underserved and disadvantaged populations in Searcy (now with a population of close to 25,000) and in Little Rock. Many of the people we serve are not insured or underinsured, migrant farm workers, or members of immigrant populations. And finally, we have a Health Mission minor, open to all Harding students. Students minoring in the topic can take courses that we have developed, such as a course on the Culture of Poverty, as well as a Global Development Program, which we co-developed. This program includes a two-week intensive global immersion experience and a course in development that covers animal husbandry, sanitation, hygiene, global health practices, organic gardening, and raising cash crops.

Most of our students are attracted to our nursing program because of our dedicated global service-learning efforts. Over 80 percent of our graduates have participated in these programs – a remarkable figure given that they are not a curriculum requirement.

In all of our global service-learning, we are foremost nurses who bring our practice to the communities we visit. And we are adamant that we must practice with a cultural sensitivity that fosters human flourishing. We acknowledge that no program of learning is perfect, and so we constantly evaluate our courses and learning activities and work to improve them.

Most important, we are keenly aware that when human beings interact, they change one another. We know that we have been forever altered by our exchanges with others on this globe.

Service-learning reminds us of the frailty of human existence. We believe that, along with our students, alumni, and practice partners, we have made a profound difference in the lives of thousands by choosing the path of learning through service. Certainly, together we have made more of an impact than any one of us could make alone. And we believe that we have helped make our students more compassionate nurses.

Exemplar 2
Global Citizenship through Nursing Education:
A Partnership Approach in Global Service-Learning
Freida Chavez

My passion for global service-learning and global citizenship has been strongly influenced by my personal background. I was born and raised in a country where one has to pay in order to get any kind of health care, where health and nursing labor are market commodities, and where nurses are for export. I witnessed my father, a physician, going to a rural area on weekends to treat folk who had no access and could not afford health care. These patients then brought their prescriptions to be filled, free of charge, at my mother's drug store, which eventually closed because it was not financially sustainable.

When I joined the Faculty of Nursing at the University of Toronto, it was inspiring to see a remarkable interest in international health among the students and faculty. Students self-organized and raised funds to go to resource-constrained countries and proudly shared their experiences as "Learning in Paradise." A number of faculty members were inspired by the students' interest and wanted to provide both practical and theoretical support to address potential concerns about academic tourism and colonial thinking, safety issues, and burdening already resource-constrained areas.

We worked on formulating guiding principles for global health partnerships, a theoretical framework to guide reflective practice, and a "health for all" agenda in building awareness of global citizenship. We relied on Crigger et al. (2006) and Nussbaum (1997), who define global citizenship in nursing as a moral responsibility to care and promote health beyond local communities and national institutions.

As part of this initiative, we developed a new course, Critical Perspectives in Global Health (NUR 480), for which students could apply upon completion of all BScN courses and clinicals. Through the framework of the course, we place students in a six-week preceptored primary health care (PHC) practicum focused on priority clinical areas identified by host agencies. NUR480 provides an opportunity for an enriched, independent experience of clinical practice in resource-constrained settings, both within Canada and internationally. Theoretically, this course is guided by a postcolonial feminist perspective. That is, we challenge assumptions of the west as the universal center, deliberately de-center the dominant culture, and give voice to marginalized people who have historically been silenced (Kirkham & Brown, 2006).

When the course was launched in 2006, we placed students in a variety of settings that offered opportunities to critically analyze the impact of poverty, power, race/ethnicity, gender, social class, nationality and other social or political issues on health. We arranged with the National Aboriginal Health Organization (NAHO), an aboriginal-controlled non-profit organization partly supported by Health Canada, to place students at two First Nations reserves in Canada: in Moose Factory, Ontario, and the Conne River in Newfoundland and Labrador. We found placements for other students in four communities abroad: Kep, Cambodia; Addis Ababa, Ethiopia; Windhoek, Namibia; and Hyderabad, India. In 2008, in order to strengthen our partnerships and build capacity and sustainability with our host organizations, we streamlined placements to the various sites.

In preparing the students for their clinical placements, we are sensitive to the fact that students want to make a contribution, but at the same time it is important not to burden our colleagues in already resource-constrained settings. Needs assessments are conducted to ensure that students' contributions are in alignment with the specific needs identified by our host partners. The preparatory seminars emphasize the importance of facilitating partnerships and empowerment in relationships with clients and colleagues. We are guided by the principles of respect, reciprocity and mutual learning, capacity building, and sustainability.

The course has three components: pre-departure preparation, placement, and post-placement debriefing and wrap-up. Pre-departure seminars are given over a six-month period and include an introduction to the postcolonial feminist perspective; a seminar on globalization; "Social justice and nursing"; "Nursing and the "Other"; and seminars on safety abroad, local health systems, and practical preparations.

As noted, placements consist of a six-week preceptored PHC practicum focused on clinical areas identified as priorities by our host agencies. Preceptors at the host agencies work with students, supported by our faculty members through electronic and telephone communication. Students keep a daily log in order to process events as they occur, and integrate relevant material into a reflective photo-journal. At the end of the program, the students write a reflective summary evaluating the program. We ask them to identify and explain situations when their assumptions have been challenged, when they felt discomfort in taking action or felt great confidence in their proposed course of action, and when they felt like a member of a minority.

Upon the students' return, they take part in a debriefing session where they discuss their learning opportunities, the challenges they experienced, and suggestions for strengthening the experience for future students. Based on these evaluations, we are currently creating a formal student-alumni-faculty network. Alumni of NUR 480 will provide an information session, aid in presenting the pre-departure seminars, and participate in the debriefing sessions. This will facilitate ongoing reflection on global citizenship in nursing, particularly for the benefit of students making the transition to novice nurses. Along with our partner organizations, we continue to explore additional strategies for capacity building, creation of professional networks, and mutual learning to ensure the sustainability of our partnerships.

References

Crigger, N, Brannigan, M., Baird,M. (2006) Compassionate nursing professionals as good-citizens of the world. *Advances in Nursing Science, 29*(1), 15-26.

Kirkham, S.R. & Browne, A.J. (2006). Toward a critical theoretical interpretation of social justice discourses in nursing. *Advances in Nursing Science, 29*(4), 324-339.

Nussbaum, M. C. (1997). *Cultivating humanity: A classical defense of reform in liberal education.* Cambridge, MA: Harvard University Press.

Exemplar 3
Nursing in Ireland Through a Student's Eyes
Amanda M. Giordano

In 2004, I was given the opportunity of a lifetime. I traveled to Ireland to learn first-hand about the things I was being taught in the classroom. I spent a month in a foreign country learning how they practiced nursing and about the cultural context. As a student, I spent my days reading textbooks and listening to lectures on how to become culturally competent. As a nurse, I need to put myself in the patient's shoes in order to provide the care they need. My month in Ireland was spent talking to nurses and practicing side by side with them. Here is a brief look at my journey and the lessons I learned.

Following the completion of my seventh semester in nursing school, I applied to an international nursing study abroad program in Ireland. I had never heard of a study abroad nursing program. I studied abroad in Argentina as part of my Spanish degree, but I could tell this was going to be different. I couldn't wait to take what I had been learning in the classroom into the world. Indeed, today I use the lessons I learned in Ireland in my everyday practice.

Our group of 14 nursing students started our journey with extensive classroom training. As a group, we considered various scenarios of what things might be like during our month abroad. These sessions took cultural sensitivity to a whole new level. It was exciting. We were researching the background behind a culture, not to write a paper and obtain a grade, but to better understand what we would experience. The more I read and learned, the more excited I got about the trip. Before I knew it, we were on a plane to Ireland ready to be immersed in the culture.

When we got to Dublin, I saw the books did not do the city justice. It was gorgeous. The buildings resonated with more history than textbooks can hold, the green rolling hills were more vibrant than the pictures suggested, and driving on the left side of the road was going to take some getting used to. There are times you learn that Americans may not be well liked. Early in our travels, an older Irish gentleman confronted us, demanding that we go back to the United States and "back to Bush." He was angry. President Bush had just visited Ireland and made a few comments that were not well received. As an American, I was automatically associated with the comments. I realized that this month was going to teach me more than any of my textbooks.

Part of our trip was spent shadowing the nurses in a small country hospital. I spent a week following a nurse in the Emergency Department. I discovered a number of differences between health care in Ireland and the U.S., but the one similarity that stood out was the overflowing waiting room. There was not an empty seat in the house. It felt like home. As I took a closer look, though, I realized that although the number of people was the same, the ailments appeared to be different. I saw arms wrapped tight with cloth bandages soaked through with blood and patients slumped over in their chairs too weak to hold themselves up. Why hadn't they come in sooner?

Our first patient was a middle-aged gentleman with his arm wrapped in a bloodstained cloth bandage. When asked about his injury, he said that he had cut his arm on a piece of farm equipment three days ago while mowing the hay. He would have come sooner but the hay had to be cut, bundled, and loaded to be sold, and he was the only one to do it. Every story was the same. I learned that the culture was work-focused and one's health was only a close second. Very few people sought medical attention for the common cold or flu virus, which I have found to be quite common in the U.S.

The gentleman with the injured arm was in need of an IV to hydrate and administer pain medications and antibiotics. In the U.S., nurses place the IVs, hang the fluids, and administer the medications. In Ireland it was the physician's responsibility to place the IV. Physicians had a few other responsibilities more common to nurses in the U.S., changing the familiar flow of a U.S. emergency department to the rhythms of Irish medicine.

Apart from the differences in medical practices, I learned the importance of Tea Time in Ireland. Whether in the hospital, on your day off, or in an all-day lecture, there were multiple opportunities for a tea break. As wonderful as the tea was, this time was really set aside to chat and catch up with colleagues, friends, or new acquaintances. On a day off, many of us attended High Tea in a historic downtown hotel. Although a special occasion for many of us, it appeared to be just another afternoon for the locals. I brought this custom home with me. I found that stopping for even a few minutes in your busy day to chat with those around you creates sort of a reset before diving back in to the hustle and bustle of the work place. To this day I drink nothing but tea.

As a bedside nurse in the U.S., we care for patients from every walk of life and from every country imaginable. Often we do not know the language or the traditional cultural practices of our patients, but we are expected to care for the needs of those patients and be sensitive to their cultural differences. In Ireland, I learned that what I may think is important, may not be a priority to others. By acknowledging these differences, I am able to put my opinions aside and provide the best possible nursing care, as I was taught in school. Cultural sensitivity is not taught in books or lectures, but rather by putting yourself in a position to experience it firsthand. So I say thank you to my nurse colleagues in Ireland for allowing me to walk in their shoes, and thank you to my teacher for bring us out of the classroom to learn one of life's most valuable lessons. Sláinte!

Exemplar 4
Timing is Everything
Jane Sumner

You might have the marvelous idea to join forces with colleagues in a school of nursing in another country. You and your fellow initiators may be bubbling with enthusiasm, absolutely sure that others will be equally excited and determined to make it work. How deflating it is when you find no support, and gradually the whole thing fizzles. This story is about such an experience, and is offered as a cautionary tale.

I work in a school of nursing in a health sciences center in a southern state in the United States. My dream has always been that colleagues would work together in a bound-ary-less, seamless world, and that our students, either undergraduate or graduate, would have an opportunity to spend a semester or part of one in another country. I thought it a wonderful opportunity to expand the minds of students. One of our associate deans was somewhat enthused, but left it to me to create the program.

I have attended national and international conferences for many years, and so have a global network of colleagues and friends. At one such conference, I met an Englishman who was professor and dean of a nursing school in the United Kingdom. We both agreed that the idea was worth exploring. He saw the same opportunities as I, and indeed his school already had a semester-long program hosting graduate students from another U.S. institution. I met with some of those students when I visited the U.K. school, and they explained what they and their school had to do to achieve the overseas experience – down to the simplest things, like having a transformer for one's laptop, so it didn't blow the first time it was used! Visiting this U.K. school reassured me that faculty members there were positive about hosting foreign students, particularly graduate students who had definite projects they wanted to complete while in the U.K. The facilities were there to make the experience work. Another member of this faculty was doing a lot of work at an Australian school of nursing at the time, flying back and forth several times a year, so the dean most certainly had knowledge and experience of what was involved.

My colleague and I carefully discussed how we could implement the dream. My then-dean agreed that it would be a wonderful opportunity for the school, and gave the go-ahead to pursue the idea. She wanted, however, to make sure we understood what was involved in planning and developing such a program. For one thing, our students would have to find their own funds for this opportunity. In retrospect, I realize the dean encouraged my enthusiasm without throwing the weight of the school behind the idea. This was an important lesson to learn: when dealing with an institution, it is crucial to understand the key administrators' style of management and to learn how to work within it. Vision and passion are fine, but not enough.

So, it seemed my dream really might come to fruition. I immediately looked carefully at both the undergraduate and graduate courses offered at our school to find out which would be best for an overseas experience. I investigated the types of experiences the students would have while abroad, who would accompany them, where would they live, and what activities outside nursing education could be part of the program. Would going to museums and historical monuments, or walking the streets of the historic cities of the U.K., be included in the credit awarded for the course and the experience? What kind of housing was available, and what would be the associated costs? Would the U.K. school provide the sort of hands-on work our students were used to in our school's clinical experiences, or would our students simply be observers? Would they sit in classes with their U.K. counterparts? What insurance would be needed and what would be our school's overall responsibility for the individual students? Would the experience be for the entire semester or only part? Regardless of length, how would the students make up content that was being taught at home for that course and semester? Would all the students in the class be able to take up this opportunity? The list seemed to go on and on, with no easy answers. I was beginning to get more than a little apprehensive. But since I am a New Zealander who had lived in the U.K. and knew it well, I thought it was doable.

The program I envisaged would also provide a wonderful opportunity for English student nurses to come to our city, and experience what we had to offer and our ways of providing nursing education. But then the same questions I had been mulling over for our students became the same questions for operationalizing the experience on our end for the visiting students. This didn't seem too overwhelming, because our medical school has a vigorous exchange program for medical students, particularly students from Germany. I knew of this program because my husband and I had entertained many of the exchange students while our son was in medical school. It could happen!

Unexpectedly, my English colleague came to visit our school. He and the associate dean immediately got along well, and that seemed to iron out some of the hurdles. My colleague's previous experience with U.S. graduate students made him confident our plan was workable. When he left to return to the U.K., both of us felt positive we were going to have an exchange.

Unfortunately, thereafter things didn't go as planned. First, regrettably, because of a breakdown in electronic communications, the contract got lost. Each of us thought the other had it, and each began to blame the other. My dean became less and less enthusiastic, and was less available to meet and discuss issues. Then, my U.K. colleague left his school to take a position in Australia! So my great idea had gone off like a damp squib, and I was left with regret and disappointment. Months of thinking and planning had been put into this project, but it just wasn't going to happen.

Another faculty member joined forces with someone in the school of social work, and they managed to take students to the U.K. one summer. However, that happened only once, then fizzled too. Yet our undergraduate students in the Christian Student Association did a short service project every summer in Central America organized by one highly motivated, committed faculty member. This was a short-term service venture that didn't involve the school in any way beyond the school's logo being on the students' lab coats. It seemed that once the school administration had to deal with credit hours and contracts, things became difficult.

I drew three lessons from this experience. First, committed support from the top is crucial. Second, do not take on a project of this size alone. There must be others on your faculty, ideally with experience of travelling abroad, who can see the vision and are willing to work with you. And finally, timing is key. Sometimes the time is just not right, and no matter how much effort you put in the project just won't get off the ground, let alone be sustained. At the time I describe, our school clearly wasn't ready for the adventure. Maybe one day it will be.

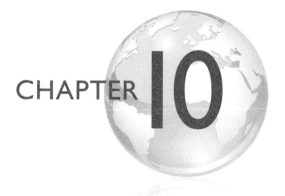

CHAPTER 10

International Service-Learning in United States
Schools of Nursing

Tamara H. McKinnon
Angela M. McNelis

Growing interest in the global perspective on health and changing United States demographics are influencing current approaches to health care education (Brown, Cueto, & Fee, 2006; Pechak & Thompson, 2009). Schools of nursing are looking for ways to provide students with the requisite skills for living and working in a global community. Increasingly, international service-learning (ISL), study abroad, and exchange programs are seen as ways to help achieve that goal. (While the terms international service-learning and global service-learning are often used interchangeably in the literature, global is a more encompassing term, covering both local and international programs. International programs are those in which participants travel to a country other than their own. This chapter – and the survey it describes – deal specifically with information relating to international programs.)

This chapter presents results of a national survey conducted by the National League for Nursing (NLN) on ISL and study abroad programs in U.S. schools of nursing. The survey represents the first study to explore the extent or types of such programs in U.S. nursing schools. We gathered data from nearly 500 U.S. nursing schools on the number and types of programs they run; student participation; types of credit available; the perceived value of the programs; the likelihood of program expansion; obstacles to program expansion; and school of nursing demographics. This information is important to nurse educators as they design programs that can prepare nurses capable of working effectively in the increasingly global work of health care.

The National Council of State Boards of Nursing (NCSBN) supports the development of nurse educators as global leaders (www.ncsbn.org). Their report on innovations in teaching (NCSBN, 2011) highlights opportunities and challenges related to integration of innovative teaching practices into schools of nursing. A unified approach to ISL as an innovative and meaningful teaching strategy is challenging, since individual states vary in their attitudes toward and procedures for approving ISL programs for credit toward fulfillment of nursing degree requirements. NCSBN is in the process of developing a survey to be sent to every state board of registered nursing regarding their policies in this regard (N. Spector, personal communication, February 11, 2011). Results from this survey will contribute to the foundational information on ISL in U.S. nursing schools.

Background and Literature Review

The growing body of literature on ISL falls into two main groups: reports on the authors' personal experiences setting up and implementing ISL programs, and studies that seek to measure outcomes of these programs for participants and communities. Following are examples of articles in both categories. (Some papers will fall into both groups.)

Observational Literature

Early reports on the development of ISL are predominantly qualitative in design and were written by researchers who were pioneers in the field. Authors provided accounts of their personal experience and analyses of literature on the topics of service-learning, methods for developing cultural competence in students, and partnerships with host communities.

In a seminal work on service-learning, Lough (1999) described an academic-community partnership in nursing. Lough's article is frequently cited in current research, as it was one of the earliest works to describe service-learning within the field of nursing. The author, a faculty member at the Marquette University College of Nursing, describes early endeavors, dating back to 1982, to engage students in service-learning activities. The need for new educational models for baccalaureate and master's level nursing preparation, anticipated new models for health care delivery, and the emerging role of the professional nurse are all cited as reasons for involving students in service-learning activities. A focus on the provision of "point-of-living" care is emphasized. Lough describes beneficial outcomes for nursing students and host programs (target communities) involved in the service-learning activity. Terms such as *partnership, point-of-living care,* and n*ew models for healthcare delivery* are as relevant today as they were over a decade ago when the article was written.

In a more recent work, Walsh (2003) reports on her experience coordinating humanitarian missions to underserved communities in Guatemala. As with Lough's account of service-learning, Walsh describes critical planning considerations such as mutual goal setting and collaborative interventions. The author describes beneficial effects of the program on participants, such as increased self-confidence and self-awareness, an expanded worldview, and enhanced teamwork capabilities.

Anderson, Calvillo and Fongwa (2007) address the issue of cultural competence enhancement in nursing school educational practices, with a focus on the community-based participatory research (CBPR) model – a method designed to involve community members, stakeholders, and research participants in decision-making related to the provision of service. The authors' research supports the value of developing genuinely collaborative programs that foster trust and respect between providers and communities. They describe enhanced cultural competence among students, providers, and faculty following program participation.

Memmott et al. (2010) examine practical considerations for ISL program development. The authors address challenges facing nursing schools as they embark on developing sustainable ISL programs. Based on their years of experience developing ISL programs in numerous countries and in culturally distinct communities throughout the U.S., Memmott et al. outline a list of recommendations on topics such as finding a fit within the mission;

selecting an appropriate model; selecting and developing faculty; developing the site; student selection; designing the course; and evaluation. The authors highlight cultural, financial, environmental, and political concerns, and offer valuable advice on matters such as negotiation with the home institution, sources of financial support for students, licensure, and liability   all critical for long-term success.

Research Aimed at Measuring Outcomes

Research designed to measure outcomes of ISL programs may focus on the benefits to community partners or (more often) to the student participants. Virtually all articles on the outcomes of ISL for student participants reference its effect on the development of cultural competence. Researchers have also examined the relationship between ISL and other student outcomes, such as critical thinking and leadership skills. In terms of methodology, correlational studies examine the relationships between these variables, while quasi-experimental research can examine causality and predictability (Bentley & Ellison, 2007; Nokes, Nickitas, Keida, & Neville, 2005). Walsh (2003), described above, is one example of a correlational study that reveals important relationships between program type and student outcomes such as cultural competence and civic engagement.

Various studies have used a mixed methods approach to discuss innovative teaching strategies in relation to international health. Dumas, Villeneuve, and Chevrier (2000) present a tool to measure outcomes from experiential learning in clinical practicum settings, including the development of critical thinking skills. Their results support the accessibility, practicality, validity, and reliability of the tool, which may be useful for nursing faculty looking to measure outcomes among their students who are involved in ISL programs.

Lee (2004) also used the mixed methods approach to investigate ISL. The study focused on a group of U.K. nursing students enrolled in a course with an international practicum component. Effects of the international clinical on students' personal and professional development along with future learning were measured. Students participating in the study reported feeling that the experience facilitated their transition from the role of student to that of qualified nurse. This study was particularly important since many schools of nursing in England have international links.

Nokes et al. (2005) examined the outcomes of service-learning on nursing students' cultural competence, critical thinking, and civic engagement. Competencies were measured using the California Critical Thinking Disposition Inventory (CCTDI); the revised version of the Inventory for Assessing the Process of Cultural Competence Among Healthcare Professionals (IAPCC-R); and an adapted version of a civic engagement instrument. Paired t tests found that after the service-learning intervention, critical thinking scores were significantly lower (t= -2.23, p=.04), particularly on the self-confidence subscale (t=2.29, p=.039). Cultural competence scores as measured by the IAPCC-R were also significantly lower (t=4.83, p=.000), though civic engagement scores were significantly higher (t=-3.54, p=.004) (p=.65). While the results were not anticipated, the authors reasoned that perhaps the decrease in self-confidence and cultural competency scores following service-learning training resulted from students' heightened insight into what remained to be learned.

Amerson (2010) used the Transcultural Self-Efficacy Tool (TSET) to evaluate perceived cultural competence and self-efficacy in 60 baccalaureate nursing students who had completed a service-learning project with local or international communities as part of a community-health course. The authors report a significant increase in both cultural competence and self-efficacy (both self-reported) following the service-learning experience. Paired-samples t tests also demonstrated a significant increase in each subscale. Means for total scores and subscale scores were calculated for each clinical section. A paired-samples t test was used to compare the pretest total score (M = 606.68, SD = 76.43) to the posttest total score (M = 719.20, SD = 65.44); the increase from pretest to posttest was significant: t(59) = -9.994, p<.001). An important finding of this analysis is the fact that the international group scored lowest in both subscores and total score on the pretest, yet scored highest in all areas on the posttest.

Larson, Ott and Miles (2010) followed a group of students who participated in an international cultural immersion course in Guatemala. Through interviews and in-vivo reflective journals, the authors assessed students' experiences at the following time periods: pre-experience, during the experience, immediately post-experience, and four to six months post-experience. The analysis identified three key themes that revealed an expanded worldview and cultural competence: navigating daily life, broadening the lens, and making a difference.

Evanson and Zust (2006) also conducted a longitudinal analysis of students' experience in an ISL program in Guatemala. Based on written narratives and focus groups two years following the experience, the authors describe the phenomenon of "bittersweet knowledge" resulting from the ISL experience. Themes evident in the experience of "bittersweet knowledge" included coming to understand, unsettled feelings and advocating for change (p.415). Data triangulation, using information from narrative comments along with focus groups, was implemented during the analysis phase.

It should be noted that nurses interested in ISL can also benefit from research on the subject emanating from fields other than nursing, including social work, occupational therapy (Hansen et al , 2007; Muñoz, 2007), physical therapy (Pechak & Thompson, 2009), and higher education (Kolb & Kolb, 2005; Smith, 2001). This literature is beyond the scope of the current chapter, but it is worth mentioning that Pechak and Thompson (2009, p. 1194) provide a chart delineating various conceptual models of ISL, along with references for each of the designated categories. This overview is meaningful for nursing and other health care disciplines, as it compares and contrasts various types of programs and offers suggestions for standardized terminology.

Strengths and Limitations of Previous Research

The studies examined for this review share insights on a relatively new area of nursing research (Memmott et al., 2010). Many draw on experiential learning theory (Kolb & Kolb, 2005) as a template (e.g., Lee, 2004; Nokes et al., 2005). Much of the research examined is strengthened by its consideration of a multidisciplinary literature, and by the use of standardized assessment tools with proven validity and reliability, such as the CCTDI (Nokes et al., 2005), IAPCC-R (Kardong-Edgren et al., 2010; Nokes et al., 2005), and the Cultural Competence Health Practitioner Assessment (CCHPA). The nursing literature could benefit from the operational definitions for terms offered by Pechak and Thompson (2009).

The use of convenience sampling methods such as snowball and network sampling, applied in most of the studies examined, have advantages and limitations. On the one hand, these methods afford researchers access to formal professional groups. On the other hand, these methods make samples less representative. In general, it is difficult to control for extraneous variables when investigating ISL. Self-selection of program participants poses a challenge to the validity of the evidence from studies examining student experiences and outcomes of ISL. Comparing groups of students that have participated in ISL with those who have not may be problematic, since ISL requires participants to have the internal and external resources necessary for program participation.

Few of the early studies use a longitudinal design. Many researchers cite the longitudinal approach as a recommendation for future studies.

As evidenced in this review of the literature, ISL is a complex and multi-faceted concept that is just beginning to be systematically studied. While research is moving forward in areas such as program development and outcomes analysis, foundational data on the number and types of ISL programs in U.S. schools of nursing is lacking. In addition, it is difficult to ascertain the degree of institutional support available to program leaders. The present study was designed to provide baseline data regarding ISL in nursing schools in the U.S.

Method

There are currently 2,775 educational institutions in the NLN database that offer at least one active nursing program. On the day the survey was launched (March 4, 2011), 1,953 valid email addresses were available (approximately 70 percent of the total). We used these addresses to send the deans, directors, or heads of each of these schools or programs an initial invitation to participate. The invitation was colorful and highly stylized. It contained a short description of the survey and a generic link to enter the survey itself, which was implemented using SNAP survey software. The invitation asked the recipients to either complete the survey themselves, or to pass it along to whoever in their faculty was most knowledgeable about any ISL or study abroad programs offered by their institution.

Measures

As noted, of the 1,953 surveys distributed, 487 were returned (about a 25 percent response rate). Respondents did not have to be members of the NLN or teaching in a program accredited by the NLN Accrediting Commission (NLNAC) to participate in the study. The initial invitation elicited only 91 responses. Out of concern that the graphical invitation might have caused the survey to be classified as spam by email filters, subsequent emails were sent in a pure text format. Follow-up email invitations were sent on March 22 and March 30, 2011. The second wave of invitations elicited 396 responses, for a final sample of 487 (about a 25 percent response rate). It is important to note that survey invitees were encouraged to respond even if their school did not currently offer ISL or study abroad programs. It is possible, however, that schools with no programs, or schools that placed a lower value on international learning experiences, were less likely to respond.

The survey contained 20 questions divided into three sections. In section 1, respondents were asked to describe the study abroad programs at their institution, including credit options available and number of students participating. They then responded to questions related to expansion of study abroad programs on a Likert scale from 1 (not at all likely) to 4 (very likely). The next set of questions asked how valued study abroad programs were by their nursing institution, school leadership, faculty and students, and were also answered on a Likert scale from 1 (not at all valued) to 4 (very valued). The final quantitative questions related to the seriousness of obstacles to expanding study abroad opportunities for nursing students. Respondents again answered using a Likert scale from 1 (not at all serious) to 4 (very serious). Following this question an open text field was available for describing other obstacles to expanding study abroad opportunities. Section 2 followed the identical format asking questions related to service-learning programs. The last section of the survey collected demographic information on participating institutions including type (e.g., Associate College, Baccalaureate College), support, and location, and a text box for any additional thoughts or comments. The survey took about 10 minutes to complete.

Findings

Sample

Respondents represented all 50 states. However, 51 percent of the respondents came from only 11 states. The states with the highest response rates were Pennsylvania ($n=35$), New York ($n=33$), Texas ($n=31$), Ohio ($n=21$), and California ($n=21$). The institutions were predominantly publicly supported (66 percent), and were distributed among urban (33 percent), rural (36 percent), suburban (20 percent), and multiple campuses/mixed settings (11 percent). Respondents came from various types of institutions, with the majority teaching at an associate degree college (43.5 percent), a vocational/technical school (16 percent), or a baccalaureate degree college (16 percent). Table 10-1 presents the percentage of responses that came from each institutional type.

Table 10-1
ISL and Study Abroad Survey Respondents: Number and Institutional Type

Institution type	n (%)
Vocational/technical school or high school	78 (16%)
Associate degree college. All degrees are at the associate level, or fewer than 10 percent of all undergraduate degrees are baccalaureate degrees.	212 (44%)
Baccalaureate college. Baccalaureate degrees represent at least 10 percent of all undergraduate degrees, and fewer than 50 master's degrees or 20 doctoral degrees are awarded each year.	78 (16%)
Master's-level college/university. Awards at least 50 master's degrees and fewer than 20 doctoral degrees per year.	42 (9%)
Doctorate-granting university. Awards at least 20 doctoral degrees per year.	35 (7%)
Special focus institution or hospital. Awards baccalaureate or higher-level degrees, and a high concentration of degrees are in a single field or set of fields (such as the health professions).	3 (<1%)
Tribal college. Is a member of the American Indian Higher Education Consortium.	2 (<1%)

ISL and Study Abroad Program Data

Regarding the data of interest, 204 institutions (42 percent) reported that they offered study abroad programs, and 122 (25 percent) offered international service-learning programs. Of those, 110 (22.6 percent of the total sample) offered both study abroad and ISL programs. Finally, 269 institutions (55 percent) offered neither type of program.

Study Abroad Programs

Of the schools offering study abroad programs, approximately 25 percent indicated that students were allowed to use that credit toward fulfillment of the nursing degree, and about 74 percent allowed it toward distribution (elective course) requirements. Participation in such programs, however, was low: 80 percent of respondents indicated that 10 percent or less of their students studied abroad. For analyses, the responses of somewhat and very likely were combined. More than half the respondents (58 percent) indicated that their schools were somewhat or very likely to be expanding their programs within the next three years, and that study abroad programs were somewhat or highly valued by their institution, school leadership, faculty, and students.

The main obstacles to expanding study abroad opportunities were related to funding. Table 10- 2 shows the perceived obstacles to expansion.

Table 10-2
Obstacles to Expanding Study Abroad Programs

Obstacle	N	M	SD
Cost of participation is too high for students	195	3.49	.604
Lack of scholarship funding and endowments from our institution	189	3.40	.682
Lack of federal funding available to students	174	3.41	.663
Cost of program administration and operation	188	3.19	.785
Not enough staff and advisors to handle more students	189	2.73	1.050
Lack of faculty interest in facilitating the transfer of course credit	181	2.20	1.046
Lack of student interest or awareness	178	2.11	.938
Parental concerns about safety and security abroad	157	2.29	.941
Not enough program space available to meet demand from students	202	3.30	1.210

Open-ended comments related to study abroad programs detailed additional obstacles or barriers to such programs. Many respondents characterized their students as older, having children to care for, and/or holding full-time jobs on top of their studies. The "lack of flexibility of the nursing curriculum to accommodate study abroad experiences" and the stress of the rigorous course work were often cited as barriers to study abroad. Both of these situations prohibited students from participating in study abroad opportunities. Difficulty establishing relationships and agreements with international partners was also frequently described, as was the lack of faculty expertise and resources to explore such partnerships. Other obstacles mentioned were a shortage of faculty generally, and a lack of interest and/or ability to free up faculty to engage in study abroad more specifically.

International Service-Learning Programs

Of the schools offering ISL programs, approximately 27 percent indicated that students were allowed to use that credit toward fulfillment of their nursing degree, and about 57 percent allowed it toward distribution (elective course) requirements. Sixteen percent allowed no credit. As was the case with study abroad, participation in ISL programs was low, with 78 percent of respondents indicating that 10 percent or less of their students took part in such programs. For analyses, the responses of somewhat and very likely were combined. Approximately 64 percent of respondents indicated that their schools were somewhat or very likely to expand their programs within the next three years, and that ISL programs were somewhat or highly valued by their institution, school leadership, faculty, and students.

Again, as with study abroad, the major obstacles to expanding participation in ISL were related to cost and lack of funding. Table 10-3 shows the perceived obstacles to expansion.

Table 10-3
Obstacles to Expanding International Service-Learning Programs

Obstacle	N	M	SD
Cost of participation is too high for students	116	3.48	.611
Lack of scholarship funding and endowments from our institution	114	3.26	.705
Lack of federal funding available to students	105	3.26	.747
Cost of program administration and operation	112	3.17	.804
Not enough staff and advisors to handle more students	114	2.73	1.016
Lack of faculty interest in facilitating the transfer of course credit	111	2.15	.965
Lack of student interest or awareness	112	2.10	.900
Parental concerns about safety and security abroad	100	2.39	.886
Not enough program space available to meet demand from students	103	2.17	.898

Open-ended comments related to ISL programs detailed additional difficulties associated with implementation and participation, many similar to those described for study abroad programs. Most notably, respondents indicated a lack of institutional support for ISL, citing insufficient faculty and resources for developing partnerships with nursing schools abroad. One respondent suggested partnering with a larger U.S. institution that did offer ISL as a way to facilitate this experience for their students. Others described their schools as "very diverse," with students from around the world, and so did not perceive ISL as offering a big advantage. Finally, concerns about safety and political unrest were described.

Discussion

Analysis of the survey results suggests that while institutions, leadership, faculty, and students appreciate the value of study abroad and international program involvement, these programs suffer from weak and insufficient support. A large majority of respondents whose institutions maintain study abroad or ISL programs (80 percent and 78 percent respectively) report that no more than 10 percent of their students take part in such programs. However, the problem seems to be not student indifference, but obstacles that keep programs small or that prevent students from taking advantage of those that exist. Support is lacking in the areas of financial backing, provision of nursing school credit for courses taken abroad, and release time and training for faculty. While most respondents envision program growth in the future, such growth will not be possible without increased funding or administrative solutions to such barriers.

The literature suggests that nursing schools would benefit from greater standardization vis-à-vis study abroad and ISL nursing programs. In particular, a universally accepted definition of terms would be helpful, as would greater consistency between programs. Finally, many institutions would benefit from better understanding of ways in which school of nursing credit can be provided for international programs.

Limitations

According to the NLN (2007), there are 683 baccalaureate and 1,000 associate degree nursing programs in the U.S. As noted above and in Table 10-1, our respondents included 212 associate degree colleges and 78 baccalaureate programs. While these figures make up 44 percent and 16 percent of our sample respectively, they represent only 21 percent of all U.S. associate degree programs and 11 percent of baccalaureate programs. Caution must be exercised based on the underrepresentation of these types of programs.

Additionally, many respondents answered returned their surveys with missing data or answered "don't know" to one or more questions. Thus, our data are incomplete in many areas.

Recommendations

At a time when many universities and schools of nursing are struggling with budget constraints, proposing the adoption of a new and costly program may be daunting. This is particularly true given the lack of clarity on the definition of terms, the fact that the benefits of international programs may not be fully appreciated by all, and the paucity of resources for leadership training and curriculum development. However, the benefits of ISL programs suggested by previous research, coupled with the present findings that most nursing schools would like to expand such programs, provide evidence that ISL is an important issue for consideration by nurse educators.

Faculty and administrators in schools of nursing must communicate and collaborate to address barriers to international program development. Securing funding for faculty and students is a priority issue. Innovative approaches such as collaborative grant writing and partnering with local hospitals to establish "sister" status with host communities may help open the doors to sources of financial support. Additionally, providing school of nursing credit for ISL programs would give students a financial incentive to participate, or at least would reduce the impact of time and money barriers.

This survey addressed issues related to ISL specifically in order to provide baseline information for exploration of the broader concept of global service-learning (GSL). Future research may build upon the ISL data collected here to explore the application of ISL principles to GSL programs – for example, working with culturally distinct populations, such as migrants and refugees, within one's own community. Research on existing programs and continued efforts to articulate program standards are important next steps in research related to GSL. Training, and possibly certification, for program leaders is also called for to help address issues such as curriculum development and development of sustainable partnerships.

References

Amerson, R. (2010). The impact of service-learning on cultural competence. *Nursing Education Perspectives, 31*(1), 18–22.

Anderson, N. L., Calvillo, E. R., & Fongwa, M. N. (2007). Community-based approaches to strengthen cultural competency in nursing education and practice. *Journal of Transcultural Nursing, 18*(1 Suppl), 49S–59S; discussion 60S–67S. doi: 18/1_suppl/49S [pii]10.1177/1043659606295567

Bentley, R., & Ellison, K. J. (2007). Increasing cultural competence in nursing through international service-learning experiences. *Nurse Educator, 32*(5), 207–211. doi: 10.1097/01.NNE.0000289385.14007.b400006223-200709000-00008 [pii]

Brown, T., Cueto, M., & Fee, E. (2006). Public health then and now: The World Health Organization and the transition from "international" to "global" public health. *American Journal of Public Health, 96*(1), 62–72.

Dumas, L., Villeneuve, J., & Chevrier, J. (2000). A tool to evaluate how to learn from experience in clinical settings. *Journal of Nursing Education, 39*(6), 251–258.

Evanson, T. A., & Zust, B. L. (2006). "Bittersweet knowledge": The long-term effects of an international experience. *Journal of Nursing Education, 45*(10), 412–419.

Hansen, A. M. W., Muñoz, J., Crist, P. A., Gupta, J., Ideishi, R. I., Primeau, L. A., & Tupé, D. (2007). Service learning: Meaningful, community-centered professional skill development for occupational therapy students. *Occupational Therapy in Health Care, 21*(1-2), 25–49.

Kardong- Edgren, S., Cason, C. L., Brennan, A. M. W., Reifsnider, E., Hummel, F., Mancini, M., & Griffin, C. (2010). Cultural competency of graduating BSN nursing students. *Nursing Education Perspectives, 31*(5), 278-285.

Kolb, A., & Kolb, D. (2005). Learning styles and learning spaces: Enhancing experiential learning in higher education. *Academy of Management Learning & Education, 4*(2), 193–212.

Larson, K. L., Ott, M., & Miles, J. M. (2010). International cultural immersion: En vivo reflections in cultural competence. *Journal of Cultural Diversity, 17*(2), 44–50.

Lee, N. (2004). The impact of international experience on student nurses' personal and professional development. *International Nursing Review, 51*(2), 113–122.

Lough, M. A. (1999). An academic-community partnership: A model of service and education. *Journal of Community Health Nursing, 16*(3), 137–149.

Memmott, R. J., Coverston, C. R., Heise, B. A., Williams, M., Maughan, E. D., Kohl, J., & Palmer, S. (2010). Practical considerations in establishing sustainable international nursing experiences. *Nursing Education Perspectives, 31*(5), 298–302.

Muñoz, J. P. (2007). Culturally responsive caring in occupational therapy. *Occupational Therapy International, 14*(4), 256–280. doi: 10.1002/oti.238

National Council of State Boards of Nursing. (2011). Report on innovations in teaching. Education Papers. Retrieved from https://www.ncsbn.org/388.htm

National League for Nursing, Nursing Education Research. (2007). Basic RN programs by type of program, region and state: 2007. Retrieved from http://www.nln.org/research/slides/topic_geography.htm

Nokes, K. M., Nickitas, D. M., Keida, R., & Neville, S. (2005). Does service-learning increase cultural competency, critical thinking, and civic engagement? *Journal of Nursing Education, 44*(2), 65–70.

Pechak, C. M., & Thompson, M. (2009). A conceptual model of optimal international service-learning and its application to global health initiatives in rehabilitation. *Physical Therapy, 89*(11), 1192–1204. doi: ptj.20080378 [pii]10.2522/ptj.20080378

Smith, M. K. (2001). David A. Kolb on experiential learning. The encyclopedia of informal education. Retrieved from http://www.infed.org/b-explrn.htm

Walsh, L. V. (2003). International service learning in midwifery and nursing education. *The Journal of Midwifery and Women's Health, 48*(6), 449–454. doi: 10.1016/j.jmwh.2003.08.011S1526952303003106 [pii]

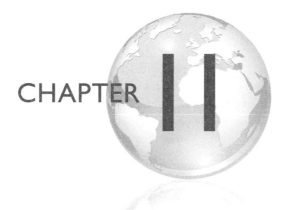

CHAPTER 11

Global Health Resources

Compiled by
Marina I. Olivieri
Suzanne Samson
Dominique Teaford

With an introduction by
M. Elaine Tagliareni

Working toward an inclusive environment and increasing cultural competence in all types of nursing education programs is consistent with the mission and core values of the National League for Nursing (NLN). Indeed, preparing an ethnically and racially diverse nursing workforce to address disparities in access to culturally competent health care services in a wide variety of settings is a critical priority for the NLN. How nursing faculty prepare students to embrace difference and to address issues of inclusion, justice, and diversity is at the core of our mandate to model professional behavior and to build a competent and socially responsive nursing workforce.

The authors of this manuscript have challenged faculty to consider global service-learning as one very significant way to achieve this mandate, and to help students experience cultural norms and traditions that may differ from their own beliefs and values. Immersion in the lives of others in a wide variety of settings provides an opportunity for students to more fully understand how individuals and communities experience and respond to health and illness, to explore what individuals and families most value in their daily lives, and to consider which aspects of their lives are most significant to maintaining function and cultural integrity.

This chapter provides a comprehensive list of organizations, agencies, and consortia that offer learning opportunities and organizational support for global service-learning. The descriptions are taken or adapted from each organization's website. Use of these resources will open the door to myriad possibilities for faculty and students to explore new approaches to cultural responsiveness and innovative options for exposing students to difference and possibility.

National League for Nursing
www.nln.org

Dedicated to excellence in nursing education, the National League for Nursing is the preferred membership organization for nurse faculty and leaders in nursing education. NLN members include nurse educators, education agencies, health care agencies, and interested members of the public. The NLN offers faculty development programs, networking opportunities, testing and assessment, nursing research grants, and public policy initiatives to its 33,000 individual and 1,200 institutional members.

Founded in 1893 as the American Society of Superintendents of Training Schools for Nurses, the National League for Nursing was the first nursing organization in the United States. Today the NLN is a renewed and relevant professional association for the twenty-first century. Cited by the American Society of Association Executives for the "will to govern well," the NLN is committed to delivering improved, enhanced, and expanded services to its members and championing the pursuit of quality nursing education for all types of nursing education programs.

The National League for Nursing, headquartered in New York City, is led by a board of governors elected at large by the membership for three-year terms. The volunteer president of the board works closely with the NLN's chief executive officer.

National League for Nursing. (2007). *About the NLN.* Retrieved from http://www.nln.org/aboutnln/index.htm

International Nursing Education Services & Accreditation (INESA)
www.nln.org/aboutnln/globaldiversity/inesa.htm

Purpose: To provide leadership in bringing together the community of nurse educators from around the world to address and influence issues related to:

• Quality nursing education including accreditation.

• Preparation and ongoing development of faculty.

• Advancement of the science of nursing education.

International Nursing Education Services & Accreditation. (2007). *About the NLN: INESA A Joint NLN/NLNAC Global Task Force.* Retrieved from http://www.nln.org/aboutnln/globaldiversity/inesa.htm

Abroad View
www.abroadview.org
www.abroadview.org/going/volunteer/colket.htm

The Abroad View Foundation is a 501(c)3 nonprofit organization that provides college students and recent graduates with opportunities for discourse and initiatives that encourage intercultural and global citizenship development. Its key activities are running the Abroad View Foundation website and producing Abroad View magazine. All Foundation activities aspire to:

• Promote education abroad, global awareness, and cross-cultural understanding

• Foster open-minded exploration and inform, challenge, and expand students' views of the cultures, environments, and conditions of the world

Abroad View Foundation. (2011). *About The Abroad View Foundation.* Retrieved from http://www.abroadview.org/about/

American Association of Colleges of Nursing

www.aacn.nche.edu

The American Association of Colleges of Nursing (AACN) is the national voice for America's baccalaureate- and higher-degree nursing education programs.

AACN's educational, research, governmental advocacy, data collection, publications, and other programs work to establish quality standards for bachelor's- and graduate-degree nursing education, assist deans and directors to implement those standards, influence the nursing profession to improve health care, and promote public support of baccalaureate and graduate education, research, and practice in nursing— the nation's largest health care profession.

American Association of Colleges of Nursing. (2011). *About AACN*. Retrieved from http://www.aacn.nche.edu/ContactUs/index.htm

American Councils for International Education (ACTR/ACELS)

www.americancouncils.org

American Councils designs programs and provides technical assistance in education for governments and development agencies throughout Eurasia and the United States and is a recognized leader in improving educational systems worldwide.

American Councils for International Education. (2011). *Educational Development Projects.* Retrieved from http://www.americancouncils.org/ edInitiatives.php

Amizade Global Service-Learning

www.amizade.org

Amizade Global Service-Learning has been empowering individuals and communities through worldwide service and learning since 1994. Over 4,000 individuals have served with local community leaders in 9 countries on 4 continents with 11 partnerships. From working with women and girls on rainwater harvesting initiatives in rural Tanzania to running at-risk youth camps in Jamaica, Amizade volunteers have transformed and been transformed. Amizade volunteers come in many forms; as students, as faculty, as activists, adventurers, philanthropists, and leaders. Young and old, volunteers have set out in partnership with Amizade and the communities we work with to serve, explore, and understand.

Amizade Global Service Learning. (2010). *About.* Retrieved from http://amizade.org/about/

Association for Community Health Improvement

www.communityhlth.org

The Association for Community Health Improvement is the premier national association for community health, community benefit, and healthy communities professionals.

We deliver education, professional development, peer networking and practical tools that help you expand your knowledge and enhance your performance in achieving community health goals.

Association for Community Health Improvement. (2006). *Association for Community Health Improvement.* Retrieved from www.communityhlth.org.

Campus Compact

www.compact.org

Campus Compact is a national coalition of more than 1,100 college and university presidents – representing some 6 million students – who are committed to fulfilling the civic purposes of higher education. As the only national higher education association dedicated solely to campus-based civic engagement, Campus Compact promotes public and community service that develops students' citizenship skills, helps campuses forge effective community partnerships, and provides resources and training for faculty seeking to integrate civic and community-based learning into the curriculum.

Campus Compact. (2011). *Who We Are.* Retrieved from http://www.compact.org/about/history-mission-vision/

Center for Global Education

www.globaled.us

www.studentsabroad.com/contents.asp

www.studentsabroad.com/cultureshock.html

The Center for Global Education promotes international education to foster cross-cultural awareness, cooperation and understanding. Living and working effectively in a global society requires learning with an international perspective.

The Center for Global Education (n.d.) *About Us* Retrieved from http://globaled.us/about.asp

Centers for Disease Control and Prevention
www.cdc.gov

Welcome to the Centers for Disease Control and Prevention. For over 60 years, CDC has been dedicated to protecting health and promoting quality of life through the prevention and control of disease, injury, and disability. We are committed to programs that reduce the health and economic consequences of the leading causes of death and disability, thereby ensuring a long, productive, healthy life for all people.

Centers for Disease Control and Prevention. (2010). *About CDC.*
Retrieved from http://www.cdc.gov/about/

Community-Campus Partnerships for Health (CCPH)
www.ccph.info

Community-Campus Partnerships for Health (CCPH) is a nonprofit organization that promotes health (broadly defined) through partnerships between communities and higher educational institutions. Founded in 1996, we are a growing network of over 2,000 communities and campuses across North America and increasingly the world that are collaborating to promote health through service-learning, community-based participatory research, broad-based coalitions and other partnership strategies. These partnerships are powerful tools for improving higher education, civic engagement and the overall health of communities.

Community-Campus Partnerships for Health. (2011). *Community-Campus Partnerships for Health: Transforming Higher Education.* Retrieved from http://www.ccph.info/

Corporation for National and Community Service
www.nationalservice.gov

The Corporation for National and Community Service is a federal agency that engages more than five million Americans in service through Senior Corps, AmeriCorps, and Learn and Serve America, and leads President Obama's national call to service initiative, United We Serve.

Corporation for National and Community Service. (2011). *About the Corporation.*
Retrieved from http://www.nationalservice.gov/about/overview/index.asp

Council on International Educational Exchange
www.ciee.org/study/index.aspx

Health issues are universal, making healthcare the domain of both the medical field and the social science disciplines. A key consideration for developing countries, public health policies are being written right now that affect the lives of millions. CIEE offers 18 programs in nine countries during the summer and academic year that put you at the forefront of the dialogue about public health and its relevant issues; introducing you to innovative educators, legislators, and grassroots organizers; urban and rural environments.

Council on International Educational Exchange. (2009). *Subjects - Public Health.* Retrieved from http://www.ciee.org/study/programs/public-health.aspx

Council on Standards for International Educational Travel
www.csiet.org
www.csiet.org/publications-resources/publications/listed-programs.html

The Council on Standards for International Educational Travel (CSIET) is a not-for-profit organization committed to quality international educational travel and exchange for youth at the high school level.

The purpose of CSIET is to identify reputable international youth exchange programs, to provide leadership and support to the exchange and educational communities so that youth are provided with meaningful and safe international exchange experiences, and to promote the importance and educational value of international youth exchange.

Council on Standards for International Educational Travel. (n.d.). *Who We Are.* Retrieved from http://www.csiet.org/about/who-we-are.html

Cross-Cultural Solutions
www.cross-culturalsolutions.org

Our Vision is of a world where people value cultures different from their own, are aware of global issues, and are empowered to effect positive change.

Our Mission is to operate volunteer programs around the world in partnership with sustainable community initiatives, bringing people together to work side by side while sharing perspectives and fostering cultural understanding. We are an international not-for-profit organization with no political or religious affiliations.

Cross-Cultural Solutions. (2011). *Cross-Cultural Solutions.* Retrieved from http://www.crossculturalsolutions.org/about/mission- vision-values.aspx

Doctors Without Borders
www.doctorswithoutborders.org

Doctors Without Borders/Médecins Sans Frontières (MSF) is an international medical humanitarian organization created by doctors and journalists in France in 1971.

Today, MSF provides aid in nearly 60 countries to people whose survival is threatened by violence, neglect, or catastrophe, primarily due to armed conflict, epidemics, malnutrition, exclusion from health care, or natural disasters. MSF provides independent, impartial assistance to those most in need. MSF reserves the right to speak out to bring attention to neglected crises, to challenge inadequacies or abuse of the aid system, and to advocate for improved medical treatments and protocols.

Doctors Without Borders. (2011). *About Us.*
Retrieved from http://www.doctorswithoutborders.org/aboutus/?ref=main-menu

EmbassyWorld.com
www.embassyworld.com

Serving the diplomatic community and the online community since 1996, EmbassyWorld is designed to provide a comprehensive list of contact resources for all of the world's diplomatic offices. Our goal is to provide an easy-to-navigate directory that is clearly laid out and fully cross-indexed. Our database is searchable via a bi-lateral search engine to search both host location and hosted embassy from dual query boxes.

It is our intention to make finding an embassy easy. Whether your intent is to travel, renew a passport, seek consulate assistance, or relocate to another nation, we aspire to provide the information you are seeking. We have maps, a growing database of tools to make variance in international standards easily convertible or accessible, as well as information on international relocation, including relocation reports.

EmbassyWorld.com. (2011). *Embassies & Consulates of the World.*
Retrieved from http://embassyworld.com/

Fund for International Service Learning
www.fisl.org

The Fund for International Service Learning (FISL) would like to help you get there! FISL is a nonprofit organization that awards scholarships to students enrolled in an international service-learning program. We understand all too well the financial strain that some students face – an obstacle that can make overseas travel seem impossible. We want to help you participate in the service-learning program of your choice by providing financial assistance. FISL offers a scholarship in the amount of $500 that can be used for any aspect of your trip: plane tickets, visas, even clothing and equipment that would be essential for the climate and geography.

Fund for International Service Learning. (n.d.). *Do You Want To Study and Serve in TIMBUKTU? TUVA? TAIWAN?* Retrieved from http://www.fisl.org/home.php

Global Alliance for Leadership in Nursing Education and Science (GANES)
www.ghdonline.org

GHDonline is the platform of Professional Virtual Communities developed and maintained by the Global Health Delivery Project (GHD).

GHDonline enables open collaboration between global health implementers and organizations in online "communities of practice" in order to create a new breadth of knowledge applicable in the field, and democratize access to critical information to improve the delivery of health care worldwide. Eight public communities focus on critical delivery challenges and are guided by expert moderators.

Global Alliance for Leadership in Nursing Education and Science. (n.d.). *About GHDonline. org.* Retrieved from http://www.ghdonline.org/about/

Global Alliance of Nursing and Midwifery
www.my.ibpinitiative.org/ganm

GANM offers you the opportunity to join Communities of Practice dedicated to:

Sharing knowledge, expertise and practical experience that build the capacity of nurses and midwives to improve health

Accessing coherent information on what works and what doesn't discussions with experts and individuals from different countries clear definitions of terminology, concepts and policy directives evidence-based tools, materials and strategies

Creating opportunities to share new knowledge, experience and lessons learned with local and international colleagues forums to ask questions, discuss issues, share opinions and work together to use our collective knowledge and experience to improve and scale up effective practices

Global Alliance of Nursing and Midwifery. (2009). *Working Together for Health Knowledge*

Exchange. Retrieved from http://my.ibpinitiative.org/ Community.aspx?c=1325c561-2b21-449e-880e-6623a1214707

Global Health Delivery Online
www.ghdonline.org

The Global Health Delivery Project aims to improve health among disadvantaged populations worldwide by systematizing the study of global health delivery and rapidly disseminating knowledge to practitioners through a range of coordinated initiatives.

Global Health Delivery Online. (n.d.). *Global Health Delivery Project.* Retrieved from http://www.ghdonline.org/

Global Health Education Consortium (GHEC)
www.globalhealtheducation.org

GHEC is a nonprofit organization committed to improving the health and human rights of underserved populations worldwide and the ability of the global workforce to meet their needs through improved education and training.

Global Health Education Consortium. (2011). *About Us.*
Retrieved from http://globalhealtheducation.org/aboutus/SitePages/Home.aspx

Global Scholarship Alliance
www.globalscholarship.net

Global Scholarship Alliance (GSA) is a social enterprise dedicated to easing the global nursing shortage, increasing sustainability in nursing, and elevating the nursing profession globally. We achieve our mission by creating sustainable international work/study programs for qualifying international nurses that include scholarships for advanced nursing degrees and practical training. As an international leader in sustainability programs for nurses, GSA and its partner institutions have funded scholarships for more than 150 international nurses. Since 2000, 98% of GSA scholars have graduated and completed their programs. Global Scholarship Alliance. (n.d.) Welcome to Global Service Alliance... Retrieved from http://www.globalscholarship.net/page/home/index.v3page

Global Service Corps
www.globalservicecorps.org

Global Service Corps' mission is to design and implement volunteer vacation and service-learning community development programs that benefit the volunteers and positively impact the communities they serve.

Global Service Corps is an international volunteer and service-learning organization that taps into the talents and generosity of its volunteer participants, staff, partners and advisors, both in the developed and developing world. GSC's programs are grounded in a philosophy that the personal lives and activities of people around the world are increasingly intertwined. It is important that we understand the interrelatedness of our individual actions and the effect they have on health, social well-being, and environmental stability worldwide. We are all responsible for the health of the world.

Global Service Corps. (2008). *The Mission of Global Service Corps.*
Retrieved from http://globalservicecorps.org/site/mission/

Habitat for Humanity
www.habitat.org

Habitat for Humanity is a nonprofit, ecumenical Christian ministry founded on the conviction that every man, woman and child should have a decent, safe and affordable place to live. We build with people in need regardless of race or religion. We welcome volunteers and supporters from all backgrounds.

Habitat for Humanity. (2011). *About Habitat for Humanity: Who we are.*
Retrieved from http://www.habitat.org/how/default.aspx

Health Volunteers Overseas
www.hvousa.org

For the past two decades, Health Volunteers Overseas (HVO) has worked to increase health care access in developing countries through clinical training and education programs in child health, primary care, trauma and rehabilitation, essential surgical care, oral health, infectious disease, nursing education and burn management. In more than 25 resource-poor nations, HVO trains, mentors and provides critical professional support to health care providers who care for the neediest populations in the most difficult of circumstances. Our goal at HVO is not only to train new health care providers, but also to encourage and to sustain current health workers so that they can continue to practice in their home countries where their skills are most urgently needed. By increasing the total number of trained health workers in high need areas, we improve access to care and the health of the world's poorest.

Health Volunteers Overseas. (2011). *Why we do what we do.*
Retrieved from http://www.hvousa.org/whoWeAre/whywedo.shtml

Heifer International
www.heifer.org

Heifer International does so much more than put food in the mouths of hungry people. Heifer helps people feed themselves.

The goal of every Heifer project is sustainability – project partners achieving self-reliance.

And year after year, as partner families "pass on the gift" of knowledge and one or more of their animals' offspring to others in need, they become links in a network of hope, dignity and self-reliance that helps hundreds of others care for themselves.

Heifer International. (n.d.). *Inside Heifer: Helping Hungry Families Feed Themselves.*
Retrieved from http://www.heifer.org/site/c.edJRKQNiFiG/b.201473/

HTH Worldwide
www.hthworldwide.com

HTH Worldwide is a leader in helping world travelers gain access to quality healthcare services all around the globe. HTH combines ongoing research, a contracted global community of physicians and hospitals, advanced Internet applications, and wide experience in international health insurance to ensure customers' health, safety and peace of mind.

HTH Worldwide. (2011). *About Us: Overview.*
Retrieved from http://www.hthworldwide.com/aboutus.html

IES Abroad
www.iesabroad.org

IES Abroad strives to provide premier study abroad programs that deliver the highest quality education while simultaneously promoting the development of interculturally-competent leaders.

Our Vision

Our vision for the future remains connected to the original IES program in 1950...a world filled with interculturally competent leaders who have both the understanding and skills to effectively, humanely, and positively navigate across different cultures, in politics, education, business, or the nonprofit sector.

IES Abroad. (2011). *About IES Abroad.*
Retrieved from https://www.iesabroad.org/IES/About_IES/aboutIES.html

International Association for Research on Service-Learning and Community Engagement
www.researchslce.org

The International Association for Research on Service-Learning and Community Engagement (IARSLCE) is an international nonprofit organization devoted to promoting research and discussion about service-learning and community engagement. The IARSLCE was launched in 2005, and incorporated in 2007.

International Association for Research on Service-learning and Community Engagement. (2010). *About Us.* Retrieved from http://www.researchslce.org/about-2/

International Council of Nurses
www.icn.ch

The International Council of Nurses (ICN) is a federation of more than 130 national nurses associations (NNAs), representing the more than 13 million nurses worldwide. Founded in 1899, ICN is the world's first and widest reaching international organization for health professionals.

Operated by nurses and leading nurses internationally, ICN works to ensure quality nursing care for all, sound health policies globally, the advancement of nursing knowledge, and the presence worldwide of a respected nursing profession and a competent and satisfied nursing workforce.

International Council of Nurses. (2010). *About ICN.*
Retrieved from http://www.icn.ch/about-icn/about-icn/

International Jobs Center
www.internationaljobs.org

The International Jobs Center and International Career Employment Weekly are managed by the Carlyle Corporation, a not-for-profit corporation whose only business is to identify and describe international career positions with employers in all sectors of the job market, around the world.

International Jobs Center. (n.d.). *About Our Organization.*
Retrieved from http://www.internationaljobs.org/aboutorg.html

International Medical Corps
www.internationalmedicalcorps.org

International Medical Corps is a global, humanitarian, nonprofit organization dedicated to saving lives and relieving suffering through health care training and relief and development programs. Established in 1984 by volunteer doctors and nurses, International Medical Corps is a private, voluntary, nonpolitical, nonsectarian organization. Its mission is to improve the quality of life through health interventions and related activities that build local capacity in underserved communities worldwide. By offering training and health care to local populations and medical assistance to people at highest risk, and with the flexibility to respond rapidly to emergency situations, International Medical Corps rehabilitates devastated health care systems and helps bring them back to self-reliance.

International Medical Corps. (2011). International Medical Corps' Mission: *From Relief to Self-Reliance.* Retrieved from http://www.internationalmedicalcorps.org/Page.aspx?pid=289

International Medical Group
www.imglobal.com

At IMG, we know that the reasons to travel abroad are many and varied—that's why our products are, too. Our full-service approach to providing international medical insurance products includes servicing vacationers, those working or living abroad for short or extended periods, people traveling frequently between countries, and those who maintain multiple countries of residence. To meet all these needs, we have developed a comprehensive range of major medical, life, dental and disability products that can be tailored to meet individual specifications.

International Medical Group. (2011). *About IMG: The Right Products and the Right Services.* Retrieved from http://www.imglobal.com/about-img.aspx

The International Partnership for Service-Learning and Leadership
www.ipsl.org

ISPL programs combine academic studies and volunteer service and full cultural immersion to give students a deeper, more meaningful study abroad experience.

The International Partnership for Service-Learning and Leadership (IPSL), founded in 1982, is a not-for-profit educational organization serving students, colleges, universities, service agencies, and related organizations around the world by fostering programs that link volunteer service to the community and academic study.

The International Partnership for Service-Learning and Leadership. (2010). *Mission and Activities: About IPSL.* Retrieved from http://www.ipsl.org/about/mission

International Service-Learning
www.islonline.org

As an international educational NGO, ISL enlists medical and educational volunteer teams for the provision of services to under-served populations in Central and South America, Mexico, the Caribbean, and Africa.

ISL provides educational opportunities for students from over a hundred universities in several countries, primarily from the United States. It is the goal of ISL to partner student and professional teams from developed countries with service opportunities in developing countries. This is accomplished by offering educational opportunities on a contractual basis to both educational institutions and individual students. The resulting financial resources are used to fund teams serving in various countries. In so doing, ISL provides annual employment for over a hundred individuals in developing countries. These jobs range from full-time employment to part-time contracts. We employ medical professionals and providers of services such as transportation, translation, guides and logistics (food, housing, etc.).

International Service Learning. (2011). *About ISL: ISL Operational Statement.* Retrieved from http://www.islonline.org/about/

International Service Learning Alliance
www.isla-serve.org

International Service Learning Alliance (Isla) offers service learning opportunities abroad for individuals to work side by side with community members who are trying to solve global problems at the local level. These partnerships provide a framework for people from different cultures and life experiences to learn from one another, discover their commonality and create a synergy that catalyzes progress.

Isla volunteers and interns work with community initiated projects focused on sustainable development. Isla programs are designed to assist communities with their worthy endeavors, provide volunteers with practical education in sustainable community development, and promote cross-cultural understanding.

International Service Learning Alliance. (2008). *Why Isla? International Service Learning Alliance (Isla).* Retrieved from http://www.isla-serve.org/why.html

International Volunteer Program
www.ivpsf.org

The Friends of the Orphans International Volunteer Program sends qualified individuals, couples and families to support the staff and children living in the homes of Nuestros Pequeños Hermanos (NPH) in Bolivia, the Dominican Republic, El Salvador, Guatemala, Haiti, Honduras, Mexico, Nicaragua and Peru.

International Volunteer Program. (n.d.). *International Volunteer Program: Purpose.* Retrieved from http://www.ivpsf.org/volunteers.html

National Council of State Boards of Nursing
www.ncsbn.org/index.htm

The National Council of State Boards of Nursing (NCSBN) provides education, service, and research through collaborative leadership to promote evidence-based regulatory excellence for patient safety and public protection.

National Council of State Boards of Nursing. (2011). *Mission and Values.* Retrieved from https://www.ncsbn.org/182.htm

National Service-Learning Clearinghouse
www.servicelearning.org

The National Service-Learning Clearinghouse (NSLC) supports the service-learning community in higher education, kindergarten through grade twelve, community-based organizations, tribal programs, and all others interested in strengthening schools and communities using service-learning.

National Service-Learning Clearinghouse. (2011). *About NSLC: America's Most Comprehensive Service-Learning Resource.* Retrieved from http://www.servicelearning.org/about-nslc

Pan American Health Organization
www.new.paho.org

The Pan American Health Organization (PAHO) is an international public health agency with more than 100 years of experience in working to improve health and living standards of the countries of the Americas. It serves as the specialized organization for health of the Inter-American System. It also serves as the Regional Office for the Americas of the World Health Organization and enjoys international recognition as part of the United Nations system.

Pan American Health Organization. (2011). *About PAHO: What is PAHO?* Retrieved from http://new.paho.org/hq/index.php?option=com_content&task=view&id=91&Itemid=220

Partners in Health (PIH)
www.pih.org

At its root, our mission is both medical and moral. It is based on solidarity, rather than charity alone. When a person in Peru, or Siberia, or rural Haiti falls ill, PIH uses all of the means at our disposal to make them well – from pressuring drug manufacturers, to lobbying policy makers, to providing medical care and social services. Whatever it takes. Just as we would do if a member of our own family – or we ourselves – were ill.

Partners in Health. (2011). *Who We Are: The PIH Vision: Whatever it takes.* Retrieved from http://www.pih.org/pages/who-we-are/)

Peace Corps
www.peacecorps.gov

The Peace Corps traces its roots and mission to 1960, when then Senator John F. Kennedy challenged students at the University of Michigan to serve their country in the cause of peace by living and working in developing countries. From that inspiration grew an agency of the federal government devoted to world peace and friendship.

Since that time, 200,000+ Peace Corps Volunteers have served in 139 host countries to work on issues ranging from AIDS education to information technology and environmental preservation.

Today's Peace Corps is more vital than ever, working in emerging and essential areas such as information technology and business development, and contributing to the President's Emergency Plan for AIDS Relief. Peace Corps Volunteers continue to help countless individuals who want to build a better life for themselves, their children, and their communities.

Peace Corps. (2011). *About Us.* Retrieved from http://www.peacecorps.gov/index. cfm?shell=about

People to People Ambassador Programs
www.peopletopeople.com

People to People Ambassador Programs offers extraordinary, life-changing educational travel opportunities for students, athletes, educators, and professionals. With nearly 50 years of experience, more than 500,000 alumni, and destinations on seven continents, People to People is the world's most recognized and respected educational travel provider.

People to People Ambassador Programs. (2011). *History and Mission of People to People Ambassador Programs.* Retrieved from http://www.peopletopeople.com/AboutUs/Pages/ default.aspx

Plexus Institute
www.plexusinstitute.org

Plexus is a nonprofit social enterprise that supports change agents in all kinds of organizations and communities. We help individuals and groups develop capacity to apply ideas about diffusion of innovation, moving from small scale experiments to large system change, self-organization and social network development. We engage in action research, provide education and training, and partner with others to design and implement high impact initiatives.

Plexus Institute. (n.d.). *Welcome to the Plexus Institute online community.* Retrieved from http://www.plexusinstitute.org/

Project Concern International
www.interaction.org/organization/project-concern-international

Project Concern International's mission is to prevent disease, improve community health, and promote sustainable development.

Project Concern International. (n.d.) *Mission Statement.* Retrieved from http://www.interaction.org/organization/project-concern-international

Projects Abroad

www.projects-abroad.org

Project Abroad is leading volunteer abroad organization. We offer a diverse range of international service projects, plus the opportunity to become part of one of our volunteer communities aboard. Our continuous presence overseas and unparalleled in-country support from our international staff ensure that your experience will be far more worthwhile and genuine than those of the average tourist.

Projects Abroad. (n.d.). *About Us.* Retrieved from http://www.projects-abroad.org/about-us/

Project Hope

www.projecthope.org

Since 1958, Project HOPE has worked to make health care available for people around the globe. We are committed to long-term sustainable health care. Our work includes educating health professionals and community health workers, strengthening health facilities, fighting diseases such as TB, HIV/AIDS and diabetes and providing humanitarian assistance through donated medicines, medical supplies and volunteer medical help.

Project Hope. (n.d.). *What We Do.* Retrieved from http://www.projecthope.org/what-we-do/

Proworld

www.proworldvolunteers.org

Our Mission: "To empower communities, promote social and economic development, conserve the environment, and cultivate educated compassionate global citizens."

In 2010, ProWorld became part of the Intrax family of programs.

Intrax is a globally-oriented company that provides a lifetime of high quality educational, work and volunteer programs that connect people and cultures. Intrax has operations in more than 100 countries worldwide and offers diverse educational and cultural programs including: high school exchange, international au pairs, language classes, volunteer opportunities, leadership programs, and work and internship placements

Retrieved from http://www.proworldvolunteers.org/about-us

Relief Web
www.reliefweb.int

ReliefWeb is your source for timely, reliable and relevant humanitarian information and analysis.

Our goal is to help you make sense of humanitarian crises worldwide. To do this, we scan the websites of international and nongovernmental organizations, governments, research institutions and the media for news, reports, press releases, appeals, policy documents, analysis and maps related to humanitarian emergencies worldwide. We then ensure the most relevant content is available on ReliefWeb, or delivered through your preferred channel (RSS, e-mail, mobile phone, Twitter or Face book).

ReliefWeb. (2010). *About ReliefWeb.* Retrieved from http://www.reliefweb.int/rw/hlp.nsf/ db900ByKey/AboutReliefWeb?Open Document

Remote Area Medical Volunteer Corps
www.ramusa.org

The Remote Area Medical® (RAM) Volunteer Corps is a nonprofit, volunteer, airborne relief corps dedicated to serving mankind by providing free health care, dental care, eye care, veterinary services, and technical and educational assistance to people in remote areas of the United States and the world.

Remote Area Medical Volunteer Organization. (2010). *Mission.*
Retrieved from http://www.ramusa.org/about/mission.htm

Rotary Club
www.rotary.org
www.rotary.org/EN/SERVICEANDFELLOWSHIP/Pages/ridefault.aspx

Rotary International is the world's first service club organization, with more than 1.2 million members in 33,000 clubs worldwide. Rotary club members are volunteers who work locally, regionally, and internationally to combat hunger, improve health and sanitation, provide education and job training, promote peace, and eradicate polio under the motto Service Above Self.

Rotary International. (2011). *About Us.*
Retrieved from http://www.rotary.org/EN/ABOUTUS/Pages/ridefault.aspx

Sigma Theta Tau International
www.nursingsociety.org

STTI, the only international nursing society worldwide, is a global community of nurse leaders with members belonging to 469 chapters who live in 86 countries. Through this network, members lead in using knowledge, scholarship, service and learning to improve the health of the world's people.

Sigma Theta Tau International. (2011). *About Us.* Retrieved from http://www.nursingsociety. org/aboutus/Pages/AboutUs.aspx

Transcultural Care
www.transculturalcare.net

Transcultural C.A.R.E. Associates is a private organization providing keynote presentations, workshops, seminars, consultations, and training focusing on clinical, administrative, research and educational issues related to cultural competence, transcultural health care & mental health.

Transcultural C.A.R.E. Associates. (2010). *No title.* Retrieved from www.transculturalcare.net

Transcultural Nursing Society
www.tcns.org

The TCNS seeks to provide nurses and other health care professionals with the knowledge base necessary to ensure cultural competence in practice, education, research, and administration.

Transcultural Nursing Society. (2011). *No title.* Retrieved from http://www.tcns.org/index.html

Travel.State.Gov
www.travel.state.gov

The State Department's Office of American Citizens Services and Crisis Management (ACS) administers the Consular Information Program, which informs the public of conditions abroad that may affect their safety and security. Country Specific Information, Travel Alerts, and Travel Warnings are vital parts of this program.

Travel.State.Gov. (n.d.). *About Us.* Retrieved from http://travel.state.gov/about/about_304.html

United Nations

www.un.org

The United Nations is an international organization founded in 1945 after the Second World War by 51 countries committed to maintaining international peace and security, developing friendly relations among nations and promoting social progress, better living standards and human rights.

United Nations. (n.d.). *UN at a Glance.* Retrieved from http://www.un.org/en/aboutun/index.shtml

United Nations Volunteers

www.unv.org

The United Nations Volunteers (UNV) program is the UN organization that contributes to peace and development through volunteerism worldwide. Volunteerism is a powerful means of engaging people in tackling development challenges, and it can transform the pace and nature of development. Volunteerism benefits both society at large and the individual volunteer by strengthening trust, solidarity and reciprocity among citizens, and by purposefully creating opportunities for participation. UNV contributes to peace and development by advocating for recognition of volunteers, working with partners to integrate volunteerism into development programming, and mobilizing an increasing number and diversity of volunteers, including experienced UN Volunteers, throughout the world. UNV embraces volunteerism as universal and inclusive, and recognizes volunteerism in its diversity as well as the values that sustain it: free will, commitment, engagement and solidarity. Based in Bonn, Germany, UNV is active in around 130 countries every year. It is represented worldwide through the offices of the United Nations Development Programme (UNDP) and reports to the UNDP Executive Board.

United Nations Volunteers. (n.d.). *About Us.* Retrieved from http://www.unv.org/about-us.html

Volunteer Louisiana

www.volunteerlouisiana.gov

The Louisiana Serve Commission, in partnership with the Louisiana Association of Volunteer Center Directors, manages the statewide online volunteer portal: volunteerlouisiana.gov. The online network connects Louisiana's citizens and out-of-state volunteers with volunteer service opportunities available in all communities throughout the state. Since the Hurricanes of 2005, the Governor's Office of Homeland Security and Emergency Preparedness has designated the Louisiana Serve Commission in the State's Emergency Operations Plan as the lead agency responsible for Spontaneous Volunteer Management in the event of a disaster or emergency. It has also designated the volunteerlouisiana.gov system to be the management system for all volunteers wanting to offer assistance in an emergency and for all service organizations requesting voluntary assistance in an emergency.

Volunteer Louisiana. (2011). *About Us.* Retrieved from http://volunteerlouisiana.gov/about

VolunteerMatch
www.volunteermatch.org

VolunteerMatch strengthens communities by making it easier for good people and good causes to connect. The organization offers a variety of online services to support a community of nonprofit, volunteer and business leaders committed to civic engagement. Our popular service welcomes millions of visitors a year and has become the preferred internet recruiting tool for more than 76,000 nonprofit organizations.

VolunteerMatch. (2011). *About Us.* Retrieved from www.volunteermatch.org/about

Washington Global Health Alliance
www.wghalliance.org

Washington State is an international leader in global health. Home to pioneering research, development expertise, and education and training, we have the resources, innovation, and commitment to improve the lives of people around the world. The Washington Global Health Alliance (WGHA) works to enhance and expand Washington's global health impact and showcase our region's role as a leading center for global health activities. Watch the video below to learn more about how global health impacts Washington's economy.

Washington Global Health Alliance. (n.d.) *About WGHA.*
Retrieved from http://www.wghalliance.org/about

World Health Organization (WHO)
www.who.int/en

WHO is the directing and coordinating authority for health within the United Nations system. It is responsible for providing leadership on global health matters, shaping the health research agenda, setting norms and standards, articulating evidence-based policy options, providing technical support to countries and monitoring and assessing health trends.

World Health Organization. (2011). *About WHO.* Retrieved from http://www.who.int/about/en/

World Health Organization Statistical Information System (WHOSIS)
www.who.int/whosis/en

The Global Health Observatory (GHO) is WHO's portal providing access to data and analyses for monitoring the global health situation. It provides critical data and analyses for key health themes, as well as direct access to the full database. The GHO presents data from all WHO programmes and provides links to supporting information.

The WHO Statistical Information System (WHOSIS) has been upgraded and incorporated into the GHO, to provide you with more data, more tools, more analysis and more reports.

World Health Organization. (2011). *Global Health Observatory (GHO)*
Retrieved from http://www.who.int/gho/en/

World Health Professions Alliance
www.whpa.org

The World Health Professions Alliance speaks for more than 26 million health care professionals worldwide, assembling essential knowledge and experience from the key health care professions in more than 130 countries. WHPA was formed in 1999 and now brings together the global organizations representing the world's dentists, nurses, pharmacists, physical therapists and physicians. We work to facilitate collaboration among the health professions and major stakeholders such as governments and international organizations, including the World Health Organization. By working in collaboration, instead of along parallel tracks, patients and health care systems benefit. Together, the partners of the WHPA include more than 600 national member organizations, making us the key point of global access to health care professionals within the five disciplines. The World Health Professions Alliance WHPA exists to improve global health and the quality of patient care.

World Health Professions Alliance. (2011). *What is the WHPA?*
Retrieved from http://www.whpa.org/whpa.htm

World Volunteer Web
www.worldvolunteerweb.org

The World Volunteer Web supports the volunteer community by serving as a global clearinghouse for information and resources linked to volunteerism that can be used for campaigning, advocacy and networking. It is an online hub where the community can meet, share resources and coordinate activities to mobilize volunteer action in support of the Millennium Development Goals.

With a constituency comprising of over 20,000 organizations and individuals, the World Volunteer Web helps to catalyze partnerships among volunteer stakeholders from all continents.

World Volunteer Web. (n.d.) *About us.*
Retrieved from http://www.worldvolunteerweb.org/tools/about-us.html

www.nightingaledeclaration.net
www.nightingaledeclaration.net

NIGH's mission is to inform and empower nurses and other health care workers and educators to become '21st Century Nightingales' — working in the local, national and global community to build a healthy world.

Nightingale Initiative for Global Health Declaration Campaign. (2009). *About NIGH.* Retrieved from http://www.nightingaledeclaration.net/nigh/

Ross, C. A. (2000). Building bridges to promote globalization in nursing: The development of a hermanamiento. *Journal of Transcultural Nursing, 11*(1), 64-67.

SigmaThetaTau. International Service Learning Task Force (website). http://www.nursingsociety.org/aboutus/Pages/governance_isitf.aspx

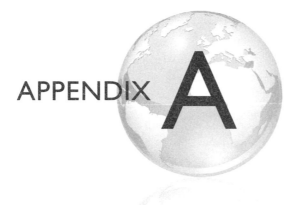

APPENDIX A

Author Profiles

Editors

Joyce J. Fitzpatrick, PhD, MBA, RN, FAAN, FNAP

Dr. Fitzpatrick is Elizabeth Brooks Ford Professor of Nursing at the Frances Payne Bolton School of Nursing, Case Western Reserve University (CWRU), in Cleveland, Ohio. She is also an adjunct professor at the Mount Sinai School of Medicine, New York, NY. Dr. Fitzpatrick holds a BSN from Georgetown University, an MS in psychiatric-mental health nursing from the Ohio State University, a PhD in nursing from New York University, and an MBA from CWRU. In 1990, she received an honorary doctorate from Georgetown University.

Dr. Fitzpatrick is widely published in nursing and health care, with over 300 publications. She was co-editor of the Annual Review of Nursing Research series, vols. 1-26, and she is editor of three peer-reviewed journals: Applied Nursing Research, Archives in Psychiatric Nursing, and Nursing Education Perspectives, the official journal of the National League for Nursing. Her most recent books, published in 2010, are Giving through Teaching: How Nurse Educators Are Changing the World (with co-editors C. Shultz and T. Aiken, published by the National League for Nursing and Springer Publishing), and Problem Solving for Better Health: A Global Perspective (with co-editors B. Smith and P. Hoyt-Hudson, published by Springer). She has received the American Journal of Nursing Book of the Year Award 18 times.

Tamara H. McKinnon, MSN, RN

Ms. McKinnon is a lecturer in community health and research at the Valley Foundation School of Nursing at San José State University in California, and is a student in the DNP program at Case Western Reserve University. Ms. McKinnon began her international work prior to completing her BSN and continues her involvement to this day. She has had extensive international experience, including volunteering with Los Niños in Tijuana, Mexico, and Project Concern International in the West Indies. She is currently collaborating with a community partner to develop a service-learning program in the West Indies, and she has led study abroad groups to Ireland since 2004. Ms. McKinnon was named Global Studies Fellow at SJSU and was the Chair of Sigma Theta Tau International's Task Force on International Service-Learning.

In 2008, Ms. McKinnon received the SJSU Provost Award for Excellence in Community Service for her work in developing and sustaining nurse-managed health centers in low-resource communities. She has served on the boards of Salud Para La Gente, a Rural Health Clinic that serves primarily migrant workers, in Watsonville, CA, and the Visiting Nurse Association (VNA) of Santa Cruz County. She worked with the Public Health Institute, a nonprofit organization in California, to develop train-the-trainer programs for the Pacific Island region. Ms. McKinnon's specialty areas include migrant health, community health leadership, and program development.

Contributing Authors

Virginia W. Adams, PhD, RN

Dr. Adams is the consultant on diversity and global initiatives for the National League for Nursing and chair of the Inaugural Steering Committee for the International Council of Nurses Education Network. In addition, she is a mentor in the Inaugural Nurse Faculty Leadership Development Program of Sigma Theta Tau International Honor Society. She served as dean and professor at the University of North Carolina Wilmington School of Nursing, and interim dean at East Tennessee State University. Dr. Adams has achieved recognition and awards for distinguished contributions to nursing education and regional engagement, including a W.K. Kellogg Foundation Community Partnerships Fellowship. She has participated in global presentations and partnership engagements in Cape Town, Durban, and Johannesburg, South Africa; Temuco and Santiago, Chile; Sao Paolo, Brazil; and in Japan, Croatia, and Malta.

Anne R. Bavier, PhD, RN, FAAN

Dr. Bavier is dean and professor of nursing at the University of Connecticut, and is also a governor-at-large of the Board of Governors of the National League for Nursing, having previously served as its secretary. Dr. Bavier has held numerous leadership positions in the U.S. government, rising to be the deputy director of the Office of Research on Women's Health in the Office of the Director of the National Institutes of Health (NIH). She created a research program focusing on nursing at the National Cancer Institute, which launched the special research supplement programs in women's health and diversity at the NIH. At the University of Connecticut she launched the first full-semester study abroad program for undergraduate nursing students that includes clinical practice experiences. Her innovative skills and ability to garner resources to advance nursing science and education resulted in her election to the American Academy of Nursing. She also received the NIH Director's Award for Excellence.

Karen R. Breitkreuz, EdD, MSN, RN, CNS

Dr. Breitkreuz, an assistant professor-in-residence at the University of Connecticut School of Nursing, earned her doctor of education degree from Columbia University's Teachers College in May 2009. Last fall she served as the School of Nursing's Cape Town, South Africa, study abroad resident director. For Dr. Breitkreuz, this was an opportunity that met two desires: to educate and expand students' horizons, and to build relationships with colleagues in other nations to better understand common issues in global health care. Between 1996 and 1998, Dr. Breitkreuz served in medical mission trips to four countries with the Operation Blessing International medical strike force, where she functioned as a pre- and post-operative recovery room pediatric nurse.

Freida Chavez, MHSc, RN

Ms. Chavez is director of the international office and senior lecturer at the Lawrence S. Bloomberg Faculty of Nursing, University of Toronto. She has held several executive leadership positions in health care and nursing education. Her special areas of focus include global citizenship in nursing education and global collaborations. She led the design and implementation of the course Critical Perspectives in Global Health, which placed students in resource-constrained settings nationally and internationally. Recently, Ms. Chavez led a successful collaboration between the University of Toronto and Brazil to foster nursing leadership and capacity building in the context of primary health care.

Catherine R. Coverston, PhD, RN

Dr. Coverston is an associate professor at the Brigham Young University College of Nursing. Dr. Coverston's research and writing has focused on women and nurses. She has actively participated in the Global Health and Human Diversity course at Brigham Young University, taking student nurses to South and Central America for six-week experiences over seven years. Throughout Dr. Coverston's education and during almost 20 years as a nursing faculty member, she has focused on quality nursing education. As associate dean she collaborated with faculty to seek solutions for several critical issues, including a path to earlier admission and graduation. She believes her motto, "Serve the Students," has enabled her to make principle-based decisions to enhance nursing education and the student experience.

Gerard M. Fealy, PhD, MEd, BNS, RGN, RPN, RNT

Dr. Fealy is an associate professor and Head of Research & Innovation at the University College Dublin (UCD) School of Nursing, Midwifery & Health Systems. A former dean and head of school at UCD, he is a UCD graduate with a bachelor's degree in nursing, a master's degree in education, and a PhD, which he obtained in 2003 with a doctoral thesis on "A history of apprenticeship nurse training in Ireland." Dr Fealy is founder and director of the UCD Irish Centre for Nursing & Midwifery History. He is also a researcher in the field of social gerontology and is a co-director of the National Centre for the Protection of Older People at UCD. He served as a member of Sigma Theta Tau International's Service Learning Task Force from 2007 to 2009.

Amanda M. Giordano, BSN, RN

Ms. Giordano is a student in the master's program in health policy at the University of California, San Francisco (UCSF) School of Nursing, where she is expected to graduate in June 2012. Amanda received her bachelor of arts degree in Spanish from Pepperdine University in 2002, and her bachelor of science in nursing from San José State University (SJSU) in 2005. While at SJSU, Amanda took part in the school's first international student-nursing program in Dublin, Ireland, with Tamara H. McKinnon. Upon completion of her BSN, she entered and completed the new graduate training program at UCSF Children's Hospital in the Intensive Care Nursery, where she has been a bedside nurse for over five years.

Doreen Harper, PhD, RN, FAAN

Dr. Harper is director of the Pan American Health Organization/World Health Organization Collaborating Center for International Nursing at the University of Alabama at Birmingham (UAB) School of Nursing, where she is also dean and holds the Fay B. Ireland Endowed Chair in Nursing. Dr. Harper's scholarly work focuses on groundbreaking academic-service partnerships for global nursing workforce development, aimed at improving access to and the quality of health care for marginalized populations. Previously, Dr. Harper served as dean of the Graduate School of Nursing at the University of Massachusetts Worcester (UMW). Dr. Harper also led the W.K. Kellogg Foundation's Community Partnerships in Graduate Medical and Nursing Education Initiative. She serves on numerous international and national advisory boards, is the recipient of honors and awards at all levels, and is regarded as an expert in interprofessional partnerships, nursing education, policy, and workforce development. Currently, Dr. Harper is leading an effort to restore, permanently display, and investigate 50 original letters of Florence Nightingale held at the UAB, in partnership with the Nightingale Initiative for Global Health.

Kathryn Stewart Hegedus, DNSc, RN

Dr. Hegedus has research/teaching interests in international nursing, caring behaviors of nurses, neonatal/perinatal nursing, nursing theory, and end-of life care. She has provided educational programs and consultation in Brazil, Canada, Hungary, and the Netherlands. She is a board member of the New Samaritan Corporation, whose mission is affordable housing, and she serves on the editorial board of the *International Journal for Human Caring*. Dr. Hegedus is a practitioner in the National Academies of Practice, and a member of Sigma Theta Tau International, the American Nurses Association, the North American Consortium of Nursing and Allied Health for International Cooperation (NACNAH), and the Consortium of Institutes of Higher Education in Health and Rehabilitation in Europe (COHEHRE). Dr. Hegedus is past President of the Eastern Nursing Research Society. She received a Fulbright Senior Specialists Award for 2008-2015 and a Fulbright Grant (January 2010) in Public/Global Health at the Arteveldehogeschool in Ghent, Belgium.

Barbara A. Heise, PhD, RN, APRN

Dr. Heise is an assistant professor at Brigham Young University College of Nursing, where she is the gerontology content expert and teaches gerontology and end-of-life care. She is an advanced practice nurse with expertise in the areas of gerontology and geropsychiatry. Dr. Heise is a member of the initial cohort of nurse educators in the National League of Nursing's LEAD Program. Dr. Heise's primary research focuses on older adults' use of personal health records for medication reconciliation; patient safety; and end-of-life care. She has assisted in establishing global service-learning opportunities for the Global Health and Human Diversity course at the Brigham Young University College of Nursing.

Marilyn Blankenship Lotas, PhD, RN

Dr. Lotas is an associate professor of nursing and associate dean for the undergraduate program at the Frances Payne Bolton School of Nursing at Case Western Reserve University. She served as a fellow in the Robert Wood Johnson Clinical Nurse Scholars program, held the Alberta Dozier Williamson Chair for Clinical Scholarship at Emory University, and received a Fulbright fellowship for 2011-2012. Dr. Lotas has been a consultant to perinatal/neonatal graduate programs in several universities, and served as program evaluator for the Children 1st Program with the Georgia Department of Public Health. She established a neonatal nurse practitioner program at the University of Texas, and chaired the group that established the PhD in Nursing program at Emory University. At Case, Dr. Lotas has developed a model to teach BSN students the principles of public health nursing and the delivery of culturally competent care to diverse populations in local, national, and international sites.

Erin D. Maughan, PhD, RN

Dr. Maughan is the coordinator of international affairs for the College of Nursing at Brigham Young University. Dr Maughan is a public health nurse who has worked with vulnerable populations for over 14 years. She has directed multiple study abroad programs for nursing students, as well as participated in several nursing humanitarian projects throughout the world. Dr. Maughan researches the impact of culturally competent education on nursing students' perspectives, and outcomes related to school health issues, targeting culturally competent care in the school setting. She has authored several articles related to these subjects.

Angela M. McNelis, PhD, RN, ANEF

Dr. McNelis, an associate professor at the Indiana University School of Nursing, has been lauded for her innovative teaching and learning strategies, nursing education research, faculty development, academic leadership, and collaborative educational, practice and community partnerships. She is a fellow of the National League for Nursing's Academy of Nursing Education, and has been honored numerous times for her excellence in teaching and research both locally and nationally. She is currently funded by the U.S. Department of Health and Human Services Health Resources and Services Administration and the National Council of State Boards of Nursing to conduct studies on improving graduate psychiatric mental health education and undergraduate clinical education, respectively.

Donna M. (Costello) Nickitas, PhD, RN, NEA-BC, CNE

Dr. Nickitas is a professor at the Hunter-Bellevue School of Nursing of Hunter College, City University of New York (CUNY), and the deputy executive officer, Doctor of Nursing Science Program at the CUNY Graduate Center. She is the former graduate specialty coordinator at Hunter-Bellevue, and she co-created the first graduate dual degree in nursing administration and public administration (MS/MPA) from Hunter College and Baruch College. Dr. Nickitas is the editor of *Nursing Economic$ – the Journal for Health Care Leaders*. She has authored and co-authored numerous articles, chapters, and books in her research areas, which include leadership and management; policy; service-learning and community engagement; and electronic vs. paper-based documentation. Dr. Nickitas was an appointed member of the 2007-2009 Sigma Theta Tau International Service Learning Task Force.

Marina I. Olivieri

Ms. Marina I. Olivieri is a senior nursing student at the Valley Foundation School of Nursing at San José State University, from where she will graduate in December 2011 with a bachelor of science degree in nursing. Ms. Olivieri has experienced great academic and personal growth throughout nursing school and is looking forward to entering the nursing profession.

Sheri Palmer, DNP, RN, CEN

Dr. Palmer is an associate teaching professor at the Brigham Young University College of Nursing. Dr. Palmer has been a professor of medical-surgical nursing for 14 years and of global health and diversity for 8 years. She has experience as course coordinator in a nursing study abroad program in Ecuador for 8 years, and she has mentored students and faculty in international nursing and course design. Dr. Palmer's scholarly activity related to international nursing includes research, publications, and presentations on topics including handwashing in the healthcare setting; frequency of Caesarean section in a large maternity hospital; retention of basic and advanced life-saving skills among international health care workers; teaching the teacher programs; malnutrition among school-aged children in Guayaquil, Ecuador; and cultural competence of nursing students.

E. Carol Polifroni, EdD, RN, NEA, CNE

Dr. Polifroni is an experienced nurse, administrator, educator, and consultant. She is the director of the pre-licensure task force in the School of Nursing at the University of Connecticut. The school's study abroad/study away options began while she was serving as interim dean. Dr. Polifroni's research is in health policy, with a focus on engaged learning, transitions from one role to another, and workplace environment issues. She is the co-editor and author of the only philosophy of science anthology in the discipline of nursing, which is used internationally throughout the world of higher education. She is also an appraiser for The Magnet Recognition Program® for the American Nurses Credentialing Center. Dr. Polifroni is noted for her leadership in academia as well as in professional organizations. She served as president of Phi Kappa Phi, a chapter of Sigma Theta Tau Mu, and the Connecticut Nurses Association. Dr. Polifroni is a frequent consultant on system- and unit-level issues within acute care settings.

Ms. Suzanne Samson, MDiv, BS

Ms. Samson is a senior nursing student at the Valley Foundation School of Nursing at San José State University. She has provided volunteer health services in Rwanda and Morocco.

Ms. Samson will be graduating in December 2011, with a bachelor of science degree in nursing. She is looking forward to a rewarding career in nursing and anticipates involvement in global health care projects.

Cathleen M. Shultz, PhD, RN, CNE, FAAN

Dr. Shultz was recruited to Harding University, in Searcy, Arkansas, to help start a nursing program that included international missions in nursing. She became the first and (thus far) only dean of the Carr College of Nursing at Harding. A leader in Arkansas nursing for over 30 years, Dr. Shultz is the only nurse to have served as president of both the Arkansas State Board of Nursing and the Arkansas Nurses Association. She has been active in Sigma Theta Tau International and was elected Secretary in 1995. She was elected to the American Academy of Nursing in 1992. Dr. Shultz has a long involvement with the National League for Nursing, having served as chair of the Accrediting Commission, the Board of Review, and several Advisory Councils, before serving as treasurer and chair of the Finance Committee from 2005 to 2007 and being elected as president-elect in 2007. Dr. Shultz was installed as the National League for Nursing president in 2009. A prolific writer, Dr. Shultz has over 100 presentations and publications, including an article in a national nursing journal with a young Arkansas lawyer named Hilary Clinton. She has received two university-wide distinguished teacher awards.

Jane Sumner, PhD, RN, APRN, BC

Dr. Sumner is a professor of nursing at the Louisiana State University School of Nursing in New Orleans. She did her diploma training in New Zealand, and her three university degrees in the U.S. Dr. Sumner teaches graduate nursing students, mainly in public health/community health nursing, but also nursing education and health care management. She is the author of a monograph, *The Moral Construct of Caring in Nursing as Communicative Action,* which presents her theory on caring in nursing. She is currently testing the instrument she developed from her theory. Dr. Sumner is on the National League for Nursing board of governors, where she serves as chair of bylaws. She also serves as the National League for Nursing Co-chair of INESA (the International Nursing Education Services & Accreditation task force), as well as board liaison to NERAC (the Nursing Education Research Advisory Council). She is on the board of the International Association for Human Caring. With her husband, she travels widely all over the world.

M. Elaine Tagliareni, EdD, RN, CNE, FAAN

Dr. Tagliareni is currently the chief program officer at the National League for Nursing. For over 20 years, Dr. Tagliareni was a professor of nursing at the Community College of Philadelphia, where she held the Independence Foundation Chair in Community Health Nursing Education. Dr. Tagliareni also served as president of the National League for Nursing from 2007 to 2009; in that position she worked to build a more diverse and educated workforce. In her role as Independence Foundation Chair, she served as president of the National Nursing Centers Consortium (NNCC) to advance state and federal health policy to include nurse-managed health centers as essential safety net providers for vulnerable populations. Dr. Tagliareni received her BSN from Georgetown University School of Nursing, a master's degree in Mental Health and Community Nursing from the University of California, San Francisco, and her doctorate from Teachers College, Columbia University.

Dominique Teaford, BSN

Ms. Teaford is a new graduate of San José State University's Valley Foundation School of Nursing in San José, California. She was privileged to be a student in Tamara H. McKinnon's community-based clinical in Santa Cruz, California, through which she learned to see the role of the nurse from a broader perspective. Inspired by this experience, Ms. Teaford pursued leadership positions as class representative and as student intern for Sigma Theta Tau International. Ms. Teaford will soon begin courses toward a master's of science degree in nursing education. She aspires to become a nurse educator and a nurse researcher in hopes of improving access to quality care.

Mary Williams, PhD, RN

Dr. Williams is an associate dean and associate professor at Brigham Young University College of Nursing, where she teaches research and evidence-based practice in the graduate program. During her tenure as associate dean over the graduate program, it has increased in national prominence, stature, and ranking. Her research interests have focused on instrument testing and development and families' response to the waiting period prior to heart transplantation. Dr. Williams has been actively involved in issues related to regulation of practice while serving on the Utah State Board of Nursing. She has been part of the research team involved in measuring and evaluating student outcomes following international and diversity clinical experiences.

Lynda Law Wilson, PhD, RN, FAAN

Dr. Wilson has a passion for global health and international nursing. She is fluent in Spanish, has led study-abroad courses to Guatemala, and has coordinated programs for international nurses visiting the U.S. Dr. Wilson spent six months as a visiting professor and Fulbright Scholar at the Catholic University of Chile School of Nursing. She is the Deputy Director of the Pan American Health Organization/World Health Organization Collaborating Center on International Nursing, and assistant dean for international affairs at the University of Alabama at Birmingham. Her research has focused on high-risk infants and parents, Latino immigrant families, evaluation of nursing education programs, identification of global health competencies for nurses, and evaluation of distance education for study coordinators at international sites. Her work has been funded by the U.S. Health Resources and Services Administration, the National Institutes of Health, the March of Dimes, and the Southern Agromedicine Institute.